SUPERIMMUNITY
for Kids

Leo Galland, M.D., with Dian Dincin Buchman, Ph.D.

SUPERIMMUNITY
for Kids

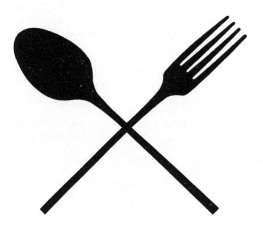

A COPESTONE PRESS, INC., BOOK

E. P. DUTTON • NEW YORK

Published in the United States by E. P. Dutton,
a division of NAL Penguin Inc.,
2 Park Avenue, New York, N.Y. 10016.

Published simultaneously in Canada
by Fitzhenry and Whiteside, Limited, Toronto.

Library of Congress Cataloging-in-Publication Data

Galland, Leo.
Superimmunity for kids.

"A Copestone Press, Inc. book."
Includes index.
1. Children—Nutrition. 2. Immunity—Nutritional
aspects. 3. Cookery. I. Buchman, Dian Dincin.
II. Title.
RJ206.G35 1988   649'.3   88-3908
ISBN 0-525-24666-5

Designed by Steven N. Stathakis

1 3 5 7 9 10 8 6 4 2

First Edition

Dedicated with love and appreciation to my family, Chris, Nicole, Jeff, Jonathan, Christopher, and Jordan. I never stop learning from each of you.

Great thanks to Signe Hammer for her help in editing the manuscript, to Carol Nostrand for her help in preparing and testing the recipes, and to Sid Baker for his wisdom and clinical pearls.

Contents

Foreword

I am proud to write the Foreword to this distinguished book because I consider it to represent the wave of the future. Certainly it is a clarion call for better nutrition for all our children. I truly believe that if even a modest portion of the people in this country would follow its suggestions, we would have a healthier and happier population.

Parents today are aware that the food a child eats influences not only his health but his behavior. They are increasingly concerned about eating, but in a different way from previous generations. In the past parents worried chiefly about *how much* a child ate, now they are interested in *what* he eats. This book provides the newest, most detailed, specific, comprehensive, and authoritative information yet available on nutrition for children. Not only does it clear up parents' confusion about the best diet for their child but it also explains when and how to use nutritional supplements sensibly to give a child's body the extra boost it needs for maximum health. With increasing threats to their well-being from chemicals in the water, pesticides on fruits and vegetables, and other pollutants, children today need all the protection they can get. This unusual book will help you provide that protection.

Most mothers do try hard to feed their families right. But all too many are still playing by old rules. All too many have been incorrectly advised by their doctors: "You don't need vitamins or food supplements. Just feed your child a balanced diet."

Many pediatricians have received scant nutritional education themselves, so they are not in a position to give parents the help they need and have a right to expect. In fact, readers will learn here that some elements of a so-called balanced diet can undermine the immune systems of their children.

The key to a healthy immune system is optimal nutrition. In this book, Dr. Galland shows parents, step by step, what optimal nutrition is and how it interacts with their infant's or child's immune system. It will be fascinating to the layman to find out that the child's immune system has to *learn* to act effectively, and when it doesn't, it may respond to harmless or useful things as if they were enemies. When this happens, an allergy develops.

Dr. Galland makes it very clear that a well-functioning immune system helps a child not only to stay healthy and ward off allergies but also to heal himself. Children do have a remarkable ability to heal themselves when they are properly nourished. Dr. Galland explains how parents can remove nutritional impediments to optimal immune function so that a child can heal as effectively as possible when illness strikes.

Many parents who have been working conscientiously to feed their families right will come to appreciate, while reading this book, that there is much more to it than they had realized. Dr. Galland makes you aware that feeding yourself and your child adequately is not a fooling-around matter. It is a very serious business and requires both knowledge and determination.

The scope of this volume is tremendous. Clear and specific advice about pregnancy is followed by invaluable recommendations about feeding the infant, toddler, school-age child, and teenager to build up resistance.

Dr. Galland also shows how nutrition affects a child's behavior. Child specialists gradually (and some reluctantly) are beginning to accept the fact that a child's behavior as well as his or her health depends to a very great degree on what his or her body is like and how it is functioning. Even in the best and happiest of surroundings a child is not going to be able to function effectively unless he is properly nourished.

Books can be exciting for many different reasons. This one is exciting because if its advice were followed it could change the eating habits and improve the health of a whole generation of children. This is a book that I shall read and reread. It is a valuable addition to anybody's library and life.

I should like to conclude with Dr. Galland's own closing statement: "Optimal nutrition in childhood is a gift that lasts a lifetime." Any parent who follows the instructions in this truly remarkable book will be in a position to give his or her child that priceless gift.

LOUISE BATES AMES
Associate Director and Co-Founder
Gesell Institute of Human Development

Preface

I have written this book in an attempt to fill the need for an up-to-date, practical, and comprehensive guide for parents who want to raise very healthy children. Sound nutrition is the key to optimum immune function. Today, most parents recognize the truth of this notion but are confused about its implementation. The popular literature on nutrition suffers from several flaws: (1) much is outdated; (2) works from academic medical centers are confined to discussions of obesity and extreme malnutrition and are of little relevance to most parents; (3) the most sensational and publicized works have little scientific merit; and (4) ideas that may work well for adults are inappropriate for children. Infants, for example, fare very poorly on low-fat diets. Toddlers are usually intolerant of high-fiber diets. And preadolescents should generally not be given large doses of vitamins even though studies in adults show beneficial effects. The most important and widespread nutritional problems among American children actually involve a deficiency of certain essential fats and the minerals required for their proper utilization in the body. This knowledge is only now beginning to extend from basic research into clinical medicine.

My interest in the science of nutrition extends back to my undergraduate studies at Harvard University twenty-five years ago. The biochemical pathways we studied were shown to be regulated by the presence of chemical co-factors. These co-factors were presented as if they were an intrinsic part of the body. In fact, we all knew that they were really nutrients, minerals and vitamins, derived from food. It seemed to me then that nutrition determined biochemistry. During my training at Bellevue Hospital I repeatedly witnessed the devastating effects of severe malnutrition on body chemistry and resistance to disease. Like most physicians, I could not relate those observations to patients who did not appear severely malnourished. When I began teaching family and community medicine and grappled with the problem of apparently normal people who did not respond as expected to medical treatment, I began to suspect that subtler forms of malnutrition might be the key. In fact, they were. My subsequent clinical research in this area substantiated my ideas and led to publications in scientific journals on the role of disturbances in fatty acid, magnesium, and protein metabolism in chronic immune disorders.

When I joined the Gesell Institute of Human Development as director of medical research, I began applying to children the nutritional lessons I had learned in treating adults. I was impressed by the similarities and the differences created by age. Children respond much faster and much more completely to nutritional therapy than do adults. The younger the child, the faster the response. I found that most chronic illness among children can be treated or ameliorated by dietary measures. More important, I realized that most of the chronic health problems that plague young and middle-aged adults could have been prevented if those adults had been properly nourished as children. But children are not just small adults. At each stage of growth your child has special needs that must be met in specific ways. That understanding gave birth to this book.

Because the most critical deficiency among American children is the dietary depletion of omega-3 essential fatty acids, Chapter 1 describes what these are, how they came to be depleted from our food, what the effects of this are, and what you, as a parent, can do about it. The key to raising children with healthy immune systems, and the core of this book, is understanding how

to provide a proper supply of dietary omega-3 essential fatty acids and the co-factor minerals and vitamins your children need to utilize them fully.

Ideally, this process starts before birth, so Chapter 2 is devoted to optimal nutrition during pregnancy. In Chapter 3, I explain why human breast milk should be the only food your baby gets for her first six months of life, and how to keep your milk as healthy as it can be. If total or even partial breast-feeding is not possible, there are ways to overcome the inevitable deficits of formula feeding, and these are outlined as well. Chapter 4 guides you through the introduction of various soft and solid foods to your child during the second six months of his life; it also surveys problems often encountered during that first year, such as feeding problems, colic, diarrhea, diaper rash, and respiratory infections and presents simple measures I and others have found effective in correcting them.

Toddlers (ages one to four) are the subject of Chapter 5, their quirks and special dietary needs. I have tried to emphasize the practical aspects of setting a lifelong pattern of sound nutrition that stresses these critical omega-3s and their mineral co-factors. Chapter 6 takes a look at the commonest toddler illnesses, such as ear infections, abdominal pain, and allergies. Its goal is to give you the methods I use in my medical practice to treat these problems nutritionally.

Chapter 7 follows your child to school, offering ideas on handling peer pressure for junk food. Healthful breakfasts, bag lunches, after-school snacks, and delicious, nutritious foods for all the holidays from Halloween to Easter are presented and described. If your child has health or behavioral problems, there's more instruction on being a medical detective and using nutrition to help her get well.

Adolescence is the theme of Chapter 8. Now that your child's diet is largely beyond your control, here are ideas for motivating him and ensuring that most of his meals are healthful. The special needs of teenagers (different for boys and for girls) are explored. Nutritional approaches to acne, obesity, fatigue, colds, flu, headache, mononucleosis, and optimum school performance are also presented.

In Chapter 9 I review the evidence that suggests that this program will not only help you to raise robust and healthy youngsters, it will help them resist the degenerative diseases of adult-hood: cancer, coronary heart disease, high blood pressure, arthritis, and other types of chronic inflammation.

In the recipes in Chapter 10, I've organized shopping hints and child-tested recipes for every meal plan in the text. There's special emphasis on creating nutritious snacks and desserts, because that's where your greatest challenge lies. The recipes were prepared with help from my family and from Carol Nostrand, author of *A Handbook for Improving Your Diet.*

I expect that most readers will want to use this as a reference book, reading each chapter when it's of use to them rather than reading the entire book cover to cover, so I have allowed a generous amount of repetition, making each chapter self-sufficient. If all your children are of school age, you won't need to read Chapters 2 through 5, but can go right from Chapter 1 to Chapter 6. Whatever your needs, you should not have to refer back and forth between chapters.

This book is primarily designed to provide preventive health advice for parents. If your child is sick, you must consult your pediatrician or family physician. If the recommendations in this book seem relevant to your child's illness, discuss them with the doctor, but do not attempt to make them a substitute for medical treatment.

I hope you will find in this book the spirit with which it was written. The most important nutrient of all is love. The nutritive superiority of human milk should be obvious to you when you read Chapter 3. But the joy of breast-feeding lies in the bonding between you and your baby. Feeding your family well in urban and suburban America is not easy. The pleasure in it comes from the love you share in taking care of each other.

LEO GALLAND, M.D.

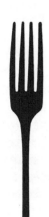

The Vital Link:
Nutrition and Your
Child's Immune System

Every mother wants a healthy child. Good health should be a birthright, and no one is more aware of that than today's new parents. You belong to the most health-conscious generation in history. You exercise, you take vitamins, and you are very aware of the importance of good nutrition. You want to raise robust children who can resist infection and disease, and who, because they are strong and healthy, will be able to use all their gifts of talent and intelligence to build successful lives.

In many ways, you are better equipped to do this than any parents ever have been. Yet, despite your best efforts, you may still, unwittingly, end up helping to weaken, rather than strengthen, your child's immune system. How? By serving foods that actually *prevent* infants and children from developing and maintaining the strong defenses that nature has designed to protect them from disease.

Children have a remarkable ability to heal themselves; doctors and medication do not prevent or cure disease. When a child is given an antibiotic for an infection, you may think it is the antibiotic that cures the infection. It isn't. It is the child's immune system. The antibiotic just makes it a bit easier, but if the immune system does not do its job, the antibiotic will be useless. When a child is unable to cure herself, a chronic illness will result. In our culture there are a number of stumbling blocks to a well-functioning immune system that creates self-healing. Many of these are the result of nutritional mistakes. What those are, and what you, as a parent, can do about them is the subject of this book.

The key to a strong, healthy immune system is optimal nutrition. But what is good nutrition? The whole field of nutrition today is full of myths and mistaken ideas. Far too many nutritional consultants are operating on the basis of theories unsupported by scientific research. Pediatricians, the main source of feeding advice to mothers, generally receive scant nutritional education themselves. And in any case, most of the principles we all learned in school are either incorrect or inappropriate to an era of ultraprocessed and manufactured foods. Old ideas about a balanced diet (like the seven food groups, now the four food groups) cannot help you provide your child with optimal nutrition. In fact, some elements of a so-called balanced diet actually undermine the immune system. In addition, your children's bodies face new threats from chemicals in tap water and pesticide residues on fruits and vegetables. Environmental pollutants destroy or deplete their bodies' stores of many essential nutrients.

So, while medicine has conquered most of the traditional childhood diseases—diphtheria, measles, chicken pox, and polio—a host of new ills has arisen to plague today's children. Allergies are on the increase, and many children are bewilderingly prone to infections—recurrent ear infections are epidemic in wintertime. Immunologic diseases, Crohn's disease (a baffling inflammation of the intestines), multiple sclerosis, and rheumatoid arthritis, formerly rare, are on the rise among adolescents.

Fortunately, enough basic research has been done to master the *new* rules of the changed nutritional game. The past decade has yielded some major breakthroughs in our understanding of the relationship between nutrition and immunity. For most of that time, including three years at the Gesell Institute, the foremost child-development center in the country, I have been in the fortunate position of being a pioneer in the clinical application of this new nutritional research.

I have written this book to show parents, step by step, exactly what optimal nutrition is and how it supports your infant's and child's immune system—and your own, as well. You will learn how to lay a good foundation for your child's developing defenses before she is born, and how to make sure that during her crucial first year of life her body builds a top-flight protective shield. Then I will take you, step by step, through all the phases of your child's development and show you how, at each stage, you can help her to safeguard and maintain her body's defenses so they, in turn, can help her mature into a healthy, vigorous adult.

The immune system is made up of an army of special cells ready to go into action on a moment's notice. Immune cells attack and destroy anything that invades the body or threatens it from within—from bacteria and viruses to cancers. A healthy immune system is always on the alert, its cells patrolling the body to nip tumors in the bud, zap the bacteria that swarm in when your child cuts her finger, and fight the viruses that give her colds and flu.

Whatever your child's age, you can apply optimal nutrition to enhance her resistance to disease, starting right now. Past mistakes *can* be remedied. It is *never* too late to help your children improve their immunity.

HOW YOU CAN ENHANCE THE DEVELOPMENT OF YOUR CHILD'S IMMUNE SYSTEM

The healthy development of your child's defense system starts with the foods *you* eat. While you are pregnant, the nutrients in the foods you eat nourish your developing fetus. The strength of your unborn baby's future defensive forces depends to a great extent on the quality of those nutrients. Your own immune system, kept healthy with essential nutrients, protects your unborn infant from most infections that may threaten you. In fact, as I show in Chapter 3, it goes on protecting her for her first three months of life.

When your baby is born, her body's defenses are not fully formed. It will take most of her first year of life before they are completely ready to begin to cope with her environment. Even then, they will need experience—they are like a newly trained army, which knows nothing of the habits of the enemy or of how to behave in combat. This is why so many infants, especially those who are not breast-fed, are susceptible to food allergies and intestinal and respiratory infections. But all of these allergies and infections are not inevitable. I will show you how to avoid or greatly reduce them.

Breast-feeding is crucial because human milk contains nutrients and special substances that can directly protect an infant against infection and against allergies. Other nutrients in breast milk help protect an infant's developing immune system as it makes its first attempts to engage its enemies, while still others help it to mature into a fully effective fighting machine. *I would strongly urge every prospective mother to plan to breast-feed her baby for at least six months—even if work necessitates supplemental feedings by care givers during the day. Breast-feeding for a year is even better.*

As a baby matures, she is introduced gradually to solid foods during the second half of her first year. These foods, her increasing activity, and the increased development of her body's defenses place new and different demands on mothers. Specific kinds of foods are important at this stage.

The toddler is forming eating habits she may maintain for life. She will begin to develop a sweet tooth, and you need to learn how to satisfy it without blocking her growing body's ability to obtain and use the nutrients its defenses need. You will learn to recognize the signs of nutritional deficiencies (which are startlingly common) and how to remedy them with foods and supplements that provide important immune-system nutrients.

School-age children face peer pressure to eat junk foods, and their lives are often so crammed with activities that they don't want to take the time to eat well. Yet good nutrition is especially crucial at this stage, because at school children are exposed to the viruses and bacteria that cause the whole range of childhood diseases, from colds and flu to German measles and strep throat. Allergies can be a problem at this age, too—and allergies are caused by an immune system that is disorganized.

Finally, the preteen and adolescent is becoming increasingly independent, while her body is going through changes that can put a strain on its defenses. At the same time, she is exposed to alcohol, drugs, and cigarettes, all of which can weaken immunity. This section will show you how to deal noncoercively with your adolescent's eating habits and problems.

ESSENTIAL FATTY ACIDS: THE SPECIAL NUTRIENTS YOUR CHILD'S IMMUNE SYSTEM NEEDS

My own research and clinical work, and the work of many other researchers and clinicians, suggests that the key to a healthy immune system is found in substances called *essential fatty acids,* or *EFAs.* You may already have read or seen on television the news that EFAs can reduce cholesterol and protect against heart disease. You may even know that fatty, cold-water fish and fish oil are a rich source of EFAs. But very few people yet realize that EFAs are crucial to the health of their own and their children's immune systems.

EFAs are essential because:
- Your child needs them to maintain health—especially to maintain her immune system.
- Your child's body can't make them. They must come from the foods she eats.

And that's where the problem starts. Our eating patterns have changed radically over the last hundred years—so much so that today we are in the midst of a famine. It's not the kind of famine that has, historically, decimated the immunity of whole nations. That kind of famine is easy to understand: it produces starvation and a critical lack of protein for the body.

The famine we face today is more subtle, a product of highly developed, mainly Western, culture. It's hard to believe, because our supermarkets are packed with fresh produce and boxes and cans of everything, but we are literally starving for essential fatty acids or EFAs.

EFAs are found in many foods, but they are most richly concentrated in the oils of certain nuts, seeds, and fish. Nuts, seeds, and beans aren't important items in the diets of most Americans. Partly because of this, and partly because we eat much less fish than we used to—and overprocess most of what we do eat—one whole group of EFAs has been virtually eliminated from our diets.

Even those of us who are careful to use vegetable oils for cooking aren't necessarily getting the EFAs we need. EFAs are fragile, easily damaged by air, high temperatures, and food processing. Most of the oil we consume today has been heavily processed.

What's more, your child's need for EFAs depends to a great extent on other factors in her diet. If she eats a lot of the wrong kinds of fats, or doesn't get enough of certain essential vitamins and minerals, for example, her body may not be able to make proper use of the EFAs she consumes. For all these reasons, we are in the midst of a nationwide epidemic of EFA deficiencies that is undermining the health of our children. That's the bad news. The good news is that you as parents can resolve this crisis in your children. You will need to follow some clear, simple guidelines offered in the pages that follow.

WHAT EFAS ARE AND EXACTLY WHERE YOU CAN FIND THEM

Most of you know that there are good and bad fats. All the media, from your morning newspaper to your evening TV news, have been telling you for years to cut down on saturated fats and eat more unsaturated fats. Saturated fats, they warn you, will clog your arteries, raise your cholesterol levels, and ultimately cause a heart attack. So you sauté or stir-fry with vegetable oil and serve margarine or one of the new spreads instead of butter. Even some fast-food outlets have switched from beef tallow to partially hydrogenated vegetable oils for deep-frying their chicken nuggets and fish fillets. This is all part of a healthy trend, right?

Wrong. To understand how the right kinds of fats can not only bolster your child's immune system but also reverse some of the damage done by the wrong kinds of fats, you need to know some more about how fats work.

Fatty acids are the chemical building blocks of fat, and they come in two varieties: saturated and unsaturated. Saturated fatty acids make a fat that is stiff and solid at room temperature such as beef fat and hard cheese. Your bodies need some saturated fatty acids, but they aren't essential—*your child's body can make all she needs.* All the saturated fatty acids she consumes are completely unnecessary. Not only do they clog up her arteries but they can interfere with her body's ability to use EFAs.

Unsaturated fatty acids make a fat that is liquid at room temperature. They make up most vegetable oils: corn, cottonseed, safflower, peanut, soy, olive, and others. Essential fatty acids are all unsaturated, but—here's the catch—*not all unsaturated fatty acids are essential.* And, as with saturated fats, your child's body can make all the nonessential unsaturated fatty acids it needs out of other foods. What's more, if she eats a lot of nonessential fatty acids, they can interfere even more than saturated fatty acids with her body's ability to use EFAs.

Unfortunately, most of the vegetable oils consumed in this country are loaded with nonessential fatty acids, many of which are created in a manufacturing process called *hydrogenation*. In order to prolong shelf life, hydrogenation converts unsaturated fats into saturated fats. If you read labels, you know how hard it is to find any food in a box, can, or package that does not list "hydrogenated vegetable oil" or, even more often, "partially hydrogenated vegetable oil" as an ingredient. Partial hydrogenation is actually worse, because it physically alters any EFAs in the oil to create *artificial* unsaturated fatty acids. These artificial fatty acids are not only unnatural and unnecessary, they can have a disastrous effect on your child's body's ability to use EFAs.

Soy oil, a perfectly good oil that when unprocessed contains useful amounts of EFAs, is usually eaten as a partially hydrogenated ingredient of manufactured foods, from cookies to spaghetti sauce. Palm oil, also frequently used in processed foods, contains saturated—that is, nonessential—fatty acids even in its natural state. It needs no hydrogenation to be harmful.

Olive oil's fatty acids are nonessential in its natural state, but it can be a good cooking oil nonetheless. It is stable, so it doesn't break down during storage or cooking to form substances that harm EFAs. It has also been shown to lower blood cholesterol levels.

The EFA Families

There are two kinds, or families, of EFAs. The *omega-6* family is found mainly in seeds grown in temperate climates—safflower, sunflower, and corn oils are all rich in omega-6 EFAs. It is also found in evening primrose oil. Because of the long-term trend toward using vegetable oils in cooking and salad dressings, most American children today get plenty of omega-6 oils—but, as we shall see, many have problems in using them.

The EFA famine among American children mainly involves the other family: *omega-3* EFAs. Only one vegetable oil is really rich in omega-3s: food-grade flaxseed oil (also known as linseed oil). Soybean, walnut, and wheat-germ oils may also contain significant amounts of omega-3s if their source plants were grown in a cold climate and if they are fresh, cold-pressed,* and not hydrogenated. Freshly ground wheat germ is a good source, too, but it is hard to get and spoils rapidly.

The other important sources of omega-3 EFAs are cod-liver oil and fresh fish—oily, cold-water fish such as salmon, tuna, mackerel, herring, and sardines. The key word here is *fresh.* Canning causes some loss of EFAs, especially if vegetable oil is added.

Both processing and cooking can destroy the EFAs in fish. In addition, many kinds of seafood popular in America—sole and flounder are good examples—aren't rich enough in EFAs to be good sources in the first place. The breaded and fried or deep-fried fillets of fish served by so many restaurants and fast-food outlets, and sold frozen in all supermarkets, contain few EFAs to start with. Worse, this method of preparation is often accomplished with the aid of partially hydrogenated vegetable oils. And frying or deep-frying, as we shall see later in this chapter, produces chemicals that harm EFAs.

There is one good, inexpensive source of both omega-6 and omega-3 EFAs: dried beans, such as Great Northern, kidney, and navy, and soybeans. A family that eats these beans regularly can meet all its EFA needs.

The foods that supply EFAs are actually the foods our bodies were designed to eat. Early humans were hunters and gatherers.

---

*An important note about oil processing: no oil is truly cold-pressed. The act of pressing generates heat; the harder or drier the seed, the more pressure needed and the more heat generated. Most commercial oils are extracted with extra heat added to enhance the extraction process. This can create high temperatures, which damage the EFAs. The best oils are those extracted without added heat ("cold-pressed"). After extraction the oil must be clarified. Unrefined oils are clarified by centrifugation and filtration. They tend to be dark and have distinctive flavors. Refined oils are extracted into hexane (gasoline). The fatty acids dissolve in the hexane, which is then boiled off. Most commercial oils are solvent-extracted with hexane to produce greater clarity, lighter color, and blander taste. Because solvent extraction removes some trace minerals, it also prolongs shelf life. Solvent extraction has little effect on the EFA content of an oil, however. Many food oils are then bleached, to further lighten color. This destroys some EFAs and naturally occurring antioxidants (see below, p. 14), such as vitamin E. Partial hydrogenation is the final step in destroying their nutritional value, as it converts EFAs to artificial, nonessential fatty acids. The oils you buy should never be bleached or hydrogenated; they should be pressed without added heat. If possible, they should be unrefined as well.

Most of the fat they ate came from seeds, nuts, and wild game. Wild game is very low in fat but rich in EFAs, including omega-3 EFAs. People living near the sea have always consumed lots of fish.

Flaxseed oil was a staple food oil all over northern Europe, from Scandinavia east to Russia, right up to World War II. And a century ago, many people were still eating a lot of cold-water fish. At one point, British laborers demanded that their employers not serve salmon for lunch more than four times a week. But overfishing has made many EFA-containing fish too expensive for regular fare today.

Without knowing anything about EFAs, your grandparents knew that cod-liver oil, a rich source of omega-3s, was a good thing to give children in the winter. Cold increases the body's need for EFAs. While they were giving it for vitamins A and D, they were also supplying a cold-weather EFA boost.

The past fifty years have been disastrous for EFAs in our diets. As traditional sources of omega-3s disappeared, industrial countries learned to hydrogenate oils, destroying the omega-3s they contained. The hydrogenization of vegetable oils has also added large quantities of nonessential fats to our diets. Fish processors fillet the fish, discard the EFA-rich organs, and replace the oil with water. And we have added large quantities of sugar to our children's diets, interfering even more with their bodies' abilities to use EFAs.

At the same time, our children's bodies are increasingly deficient in certain minerals and vitamins that are necessary to help them process and use EFAs. And the ever-growing numbers of chemical pollutants in our food, water, and air, together with such pervasive cooking methods as deep-frying, are promoting the destruction of the EFAs in our children's bodies.

To understand how these different factors have brought us to the brink of an EFA disaster—and to understand how you can pull your children out of it—you need to know something about how your child's body uses EFAs.

THE PROSTAGLANDIN CONNECTION

In each of the two main families of essential fatty acids, there is one particularly important acid: In the omega-6 family it is *linoleic acid,* or *LA*. In the omega-3 family it is *linolenic acid,* or *LNA*. But neither of these acids is, by itself, of any use to your child's body—both must be converted into other chemical forms. The body does this through a series of chemical reactions, regulated by different enzymes, that is called metabolism.

To do their job of regulating EFA metabolism properly, enzymes depend on the presence of certain key *co-factor* vitamins—B-6, A, C, and E—and minerals—magnesium, zinc, copper, and selenium. If your child gets a good supply of all these vitamins and minerals, her body will metabolize LA and LNA into a special group of hormonelike substances called *prostaglandins*. Among other things, prostaglandins seem to regulate the activity of the white blood cells in her immune system, the *T-cells* and *B-cells*, for instance, which are the major classes of lymphocytes.

These cells are divided, rather like an army, into specialists with different areas of responsibility. *Macrophages* patrol the bloodstream looking for both microbial invaders and debris, which they clean up. (*Macrophage* means literally "large eater.") If a macrophage does encounter a bacterium, it takes an antigen molecule from it and carries it around until it meets a helper *T-cell*.

The cells that give the orders are the T-cells: *Helper T-cells* send the *killer T-cells* and the B-cells into action. B-cells, once prodded into action by the helper T-cells, produce *antibodies*, while *suppressor T-cells* issue cease-fire orders when the battle is won.

B-cells and T-cells are the mind of the immune system, and they are unique. They are the only cells in the body, besides brain cells, that have memory. *Lymphocytes learn and remember who is a friend and who is an enemy.*

An infant's and small child's immune system may have marshaled its army, but, as I pointed out earlier, it is an ignorant army. It has not yet been challenged. It knows who its friends are—the body it inhabits, the foods that come into that body, and the good bacteria that help the body work. But it is meeting enemies for the first time. For each new enemy, it must figure out the right antibody, and the right response for its disease-fighting cells. That's where the lymphocytes come in. B-cells learn how to make antibodies for every one of the thousands of different germs, toxins, fungi, bacteria, viruses, and parasites that invade the body in the course of a lifetime. T-cells remember every invader so that each time they come across it, they can instantly order out the troops. A specific germ may make some headway the first time, but the second time it invades, the army will be ready.

The immune system's army works as a team, and, like any other team, it depends on a constant exchange of information, or signals, among its members. The T-cells are the key to that communication. Their state of health is critical, because they make decisions and give orders. Their ability to do that may depend, in turn, on the right supplies of prostaglandins. Experiments with animals have shown that when prostaglandin production goes awry, it is the T-cells that are most disastrously affected. And when they can't do their jobs, the whole immune system malfunctions.

If something goes wrong with her body's production of prostaglandins, then—if not enough of one, or too much of another, is made—your child's defenses may well be crippled. The result may be disease.

Your child's body makes fifty different prostaglandins. Problems in their production can be detected behind a host of twentieth-century illnesses, including cancer, asthma, and other allergies, and autoimmune diseases such as lupus and rheumatoid arthritis.

When treating a child with what I suspect might be a prostaglandin imbalance, the first thing I look for is whether she is getting enough EFAs. But suppose she is eating plenty of foods that contain both LA and LNA? The next culprit I look for is a deficiency in the key co-factor vitamins and minerals that make it possible for enzymes to regulate the metabolism of LA and LNA. These, you will recall, are vitamins B-6, A, C, and E, and the minerals magnesium, zinc, copper, and selenium. If a child's diet is deficient in even one of these co-factor nutrients, it will have the same effect as an EFA deficiency. In my medical practice, I see this over and over.

It is no accident that the foods that are naturally rich in EFAs are also naturally rich in the EFA co-factor nutrients. Nuts, seeds, and beans are excellent sources of magnesium, copper, zinc, and vitamins E and B-6. Seafood is a rich source of all the minerals. If fresh vegetables are added for vitamins A and C, we have a balanced, EFA-strong diet that can't be beat for its immune-building effect.

Unfortunately, American children today get most of their

calories from sugar, processed cereal grains such as wheat and corn, processed oils, dairy products, and fatty meats. It's no wonder that most children today consume less than two-thirds of the Recommended Dietary Allowance (RDA) of magnesium, vitamin B-6, and copper.

Zinc and vitamin A deficiencies are very common, too. A zinc deficiency is most likely to occur in the young child who gets most of her nutrition from milk and cheese. Vitamin A deficiencies most often show up in adolescents who live on meat, potatoes, and fast foods, and who shun vegetables and eggs.

If a child's diet is rich in sources of both EFAs and the co-factor nutrients but she still shows signs of an EFA deficiency, then the culprit will almost always be *anti-nutrients,* the bane of every nutrition-conscious parent. Anti-nutrients are foods or substances that not only have little or no nutritional value but also block or make EFA metabolism go awry. The list of these villains in the American diet is far too long:

Nonessential Fatty Acids. Major anti-nutrients, they confuse the enzymes that regulate EFA metabolism into metabolizing them instead of the EFAs. Topping the whole list are partially hydrogenated vegetable oils, which interfere with the enzyme action. Unlike sugar, which fills what some scientists think may be a biological need for sweetness, these artificial fats fill no human need.

Sugar. Large quantities weaken the enzymes of EFA metabolism. Sugar supplies 25 to 35 percent of the calories consumed by most American children, but brings with it none of the vitamins and minerals needed for EFA metabolism or for energy. If a child eats whole wheat bread, she gets with it the B vitamins and magnesium needed both to convert the bread into energy and as co-factor nutrients. These are naturally present in whole wheat. But if she eats candy, or a white-flour pastry, she has to get those B vitamins and minerals from some other food.

Recent studies in both animals and humans have shown that sugar increases the adverse effects of a copper deficiency, although the mechanism hasn't been discovered yet. Sugar also increases the amounts of magnesium and other important minerals that are excreted in the urine.[1]

Sodium. Common salt, sodium chloride, is naturally present in many foods. The amount found in unprocessed foods is enough for children living in temperate or cold climates. But large amounts of salt are used in processing foods: American children eat *three or more times* as much sodium as they need. This not only contributes to the development of high blood pressure, it also increases the amounts of magnesium, a co-factor nutrient, and potassium that are lost in the urine. This constant depletion means that children have to get much more of these two key minerals in their food or in supplements.

Phosphates. Phosphorus, like sodium, is an essential mineral, but, also like sodium, American children get far too much of it. Phosphates are used as preservatives in many foods, and phosphoric acid is used to keep soft drinks bubbly. Meat is naturally rich in phosphates. Large amounts of phosphorus in the system act as a kind of intestinal sludge, blocking the absorption of calcium and magnesium, both of which are important for many other reasons besides their crucial roles as co-factor nutrients in EFA metabolism.

Pesticides. These are sprayed on fruits, vegetables, and grains to kill insects and fungi, and their residues remain in or on these foods when you eat them. Some herbicides that contaminate agricultural produce interfere with the body's ability to use vitamin B-6, which means that more of this co-factor vitamin must be provided in foods or supplements.[2] Vitamin B-6 deficiency not only interferes with EFA metabolism, it may also have neurological effects ranging from epileptic seizures to a feeling of pins and needles in the hands.

Free Radicals. Your child's cells use oxygen to burn food for energy and to burn away germs and foreign chemicals, such as pesticides. This process of combustion creates tiny bonfires in the cells, and these fires give off "sparks" that can start fires in undesirable places, damaging cell membranes and destroying EFAs. The chemical name for these sparks is *free radicals.*

Frying foods in oil creates free radicals when high heat damages the oil. Fast-food restaurants keep cooking oil bubbling all day to deep-fry potatoes, fish, and chicken, worsening the damage by the hour. Your children eat the free radicals with their French fries and chicken nuggets, and the heat-damaged oils create more free radicals in their bodies.

Fortunately, the body has a "fire department" to snuff these sparks before they start too many fires. This band of free-radical quenchers is called the *antioxidant defense system*. The antioxidant defense system depends for its effectiveness on a number of vitamins and minerals, particularly vitamins A, C, E, B-2, and B-3 and the minerals zinc, copper, manganese, and sulfur. Exposure to environmental pollutants such as pesticides in foods increases your child's need for these antioxidants, especially for vitamins C and E, both of which are destroyed in the firefighting process.[3]

Antioxidants are crucial to your child's immune system, too. When white blood cells kill germs, they generate enormous amounts of heat, turning into tiny furnaces. They need a generous supply of antioxidants to keep them from literally burning themselves up within your child's body.

So your child needs antioxidants to protect both her EFAs and the individual cells of her immune system. Heat-damaged oils and pollutants in food and the environment dramatically increase her need for these key vitamins and minerals.

HOW THE IMMUNE SYSTEM CAN MALFUNCTION TO CREATE ALLERGIES AND AUTOIMMUNE DISEASES

The unborn infant's developing immune system is learning how to recognize "me"—the infant's own body and everything that belongs in it. A perfectly functioning immune system learns and remembers that it should not attack anything that is "me." Once it learns that, it can concentrate its energies on attacking everything that is "not me."

But sometimes something goes wrong, and a person's immune system responds to harmless or useful things as if they were enemies; it reacts, say, to a piece of bread as if it were a virus, or responds to the body's own thyroid gland as if it were a cancer. When the immune system attacks harmless or even useful things that enter the body from outside, whether food or plant spores, we call it an *allergy*. When the immune system attacks the body it inhabits, an autoimmune disease develops.

In my practice, I see many children with allergic illnesses, and in most cases, EFA deficiency plays an important role. Jason's story is one dramatic example.

At twelve, Jason had many food and pollen allergies. He was also hyperactive and displayed two signals of EFA deficiency: he was always thirsty and his skin was very dry. I enriched Jason's diet with safflower oil, a polyunsaturated oil rich in EFAs, and cut down on the amount of sugar he consumed. Almost immediately, he became less thirsty and his skin soon became soft and shiny. More important, he calmed down and his food allergies disappeared.

The LA in the safflower oil allowed Jason to increase his output of *prostaglandin E_1*, or *PGE_1*. PGE_1 is a natural suppressor of allergic reactions and a hormonal regulator of the nervous system; so in addition to curing Jay's allergies, it cured his hyperactivity. (Many prostaglandins do two or more jobs; thus when you bolster your child's immune system, you are also contributing to the healthy regulation of her nervous system, her heart and blood vessels, and her glandular system.)

My research shows that people who have allergies need more EFAs than people who don't.[4] The reason seems to be that in people with allergies one of the enzymes involved in EFA metabolism is weakened or doesn't function properly. Drs. David Horrobin and Mehar Manku of the Efamol Research Institute in Nova Scotia have found that in children with allergic eczema and asthma, the first step in making PGE_1—the conversion of LA to an intermediate fatty acid known as GLA—is blocked.[5] Dr. Ross Rocklin of Tufts University has found a similar block in people with simple hay fever.[6]

Although the weakness of this enzyme is undoubtedly inherited, the condition is made worse by a deficiency of EFAs. The good news is that it can be overcome by adding enough EFAs to the diet.

We shall explore the question of allergies in more detail in Chapters 6 and 9. Here I want to point out that *even when an infant inherits a predisposition for allergies, special protective elements found in breast milk, together with EFAs, can delay the onset of allergic illness and greatly reduce its severity.*

As I will discuss throughout this book, proper EFA intake is also helpful to children who suffer from recurrent infections, which frequently go along with allergies.

Autoimmune diseases aren't common in young children, but they are appearing with increasing frequency in adolescents. Diabetes, Crohn's disease, ulcerative colitis, systemic lupus, and juvenile rheumatoid arthritis are, sadly, striking more and more young people between the ages of twelve and twenty-one. In many cases, it appears that unbalanced prostaglandin synthesis, in which certain harmful prostaglandins are produced in excess, plays an important role in the development of the illness.

Feeding fish oils to experimental animals has been shown to prevent the development of autoimmune diseases similar to lupus, multiple sclerosis, and rheumatoid arthritis. I find EFA supplements empirically useful in treating children with established autoimmune disorders.

THE SIGNS OF EFA DEFICIENCY

In addition to their crucial role in regulating the immune system, EFAs are a vital component of all your body's membranes—from the membrane around each cell, which allows it to function properly, to your skin, your body's outer membrane. Because your skin's outermost layer is composed of cell membranes and protein, an EFA deficiency produces dry, scaly skin.

A healthy child has lustrous skin, and hair that reflects light without the aid of conditioners and oils. (Hair is really an appendage of the skin. It is made of protein derived from cell membrane, and its condition closely reflects that of the skin.) Few children have such hair and skin today. Instead, varying degrees of dryness are the rule—from a flat dullness (referred to as a "mat finish" by Sid Baker of the Gesell Institute) to visible scaling and roughness.

There is an easy way to tell whether your child's dry skin is caused by an EFA deficiency: Increase her omega-3 intake by following the guidelines in this book. The chances are her hair and skin will soon acquire their own luster. (If you have the same problems, or if your nails are brittle or you sometimes get tiny lumps, like a rash, on the backs of your arms, you can try the same test on yourself.)

Most experts agree that this kind of *functional test*—in

which you give increasing doses of a particular nutrient to see how a specific condition changes—is the only accurate way to assess a person's nutritional status. It is the basis for my own and other specialists' work with nutritionally deficient patients.

HOW TO MAKE SURE YOUR CHILD GETS ENOUGH EFAs

Throughout this book there will be guidelines to help you make sure your child gets the EFAs she needs. The key is a balanced intake of fatty acids, and the best way to do this is through food.

As we have shown, good dietary sources of EFAs are nuts, seeds, beans, and some fish. EFA requirements vary somewhat with climate. To maintain a relationship between omega-3s and omega-6s suitable for most people living in the United States, the best nuts are English walnuts, the best seed is flaxseed, and the best beans are navy, kidney, and soy. The best fish are fresh salmon, tuna, mackerel, bluefish, sardines, or herring.

But it is clearly not practical to expect you to ensure that your children get three servings each week of fresh salmon or tuna, plus plenty of English walnuts, flaxseed, and beans. For the vast majority of parents, food oils are the best and most practical way to supply EFAs to their children.

Flaxseed Oil. For most children, the best oil is food-grade flaxseed oil. It contains a mixture of omega-3s and omega-6s, with the 3s predominating. I prefer it because the EFAs it contains are in a form that gives a child's body better control over EFA metabolism than do those in other oils, and because of its bland taste.

Recently, a Canadian company, Omega Nutrition, has begun marketing flaxseed oil in this country. This is a superior product, unrefined and labeled with the date of pressing. It will keep for up to two months in the refrigerator. It can also be kept frozen—it won't solidify because it is pure polyunsaturated fat—for four months. If you have trouble finding flaxseed oil in stores, you can order it from: Omega Nutrition, 165–810 West Broadway, Vancouver, British Columbia V5ZYC9, or Allergy Resources, Box 2131, Port Washington, N.Y. 11050.

Freshly pressed flaxseed oil is slightly sweet. Usually, the flaxseed oil you buy will have almost no taste. *If it tastes even slightly bitter, it is rancid; throw it out.* (Under no circumstances buy the linseed oil that is made from flaxseeds, used in paint stores; it is poisonous.)

Some people, even quite young children, have no difficulty swallowing a tablespoon of flaxseed oil right before eating or before drinking a glass of juice. If there is any problem with this, you can stir flaxseed oil into orange juice (stir hard and drink immediately—the oil forms a suspension and will separate out quickly).

You can use flaxseed oil as a dressing on hot vegetables or pasta or in salad dressing. For flavor, mix half and half with olive oil.

Other salad dressings you can make are mayonnaise made with flaxseed oil, and flaxseed oil blended with yogurt or soft tofu and flavored with herbs.

For some spreads, mix flaxseed oil half and half with butter— this is better than all the substitute spreads on the market, including margarine. (Margarine is made of partially hydrogenated vegetable oil, an arch anti-nutrient.) Flaxseed oil can also be mixed with yogurt and flavored with sugar-free jam or apple butter.

Finally, you can mix a tablespoon of flaxseed oil into a health shake (see Chapter 10).

Don't use flaxseed oil for frying or sautéing, since high heat plus oxygen destroys its EFAs. It can, however, be used in baking, because EFAs don't get destroyed in this kind of cooking process (see Chapter 10).

Flaxseed oil is absorbed through the skin, and I sometimes recommend rubbing it on the skin of infants, but it smells slightly fishy.

Flaxseed oil is the very best source of EFA omega-3s. If it is unavailable, you can substitute 2 tablespoons of walnut oil for 1 tablespoon of flaxseed oil. Unfortunately, walnut oil is expensive. You may also substitute 1 teaspoon of cod-liver oil for 1 tablespoon of flaxseed oil.

Cod-Liver Oil. A fine source of omega-3s, vitamin A, and vitamin D, but these vitamins can be toxic in large amounts, and I never administer more than 1 teaspoon of cod-liver oil a day to young children, or 1 tablespoon to adolescents. Taste is a problem, even when the cod-liver oil is mixed into juice. Flavored cod-liver oil is available, and you may find this more palatable. Never use defatted cod-liver oil. Taking the fat out makes cod-liver oil taste better, but it also removes its nutritive value.

Fish-Oil Extracts. These are marketed in capsules under brand names such as MaxEPA and Efamol Marine, both of which can be found at health-food stores.

I find fish-oil extracts useful in treating diseases associated with EFA deficiency, but I don't recommend them for preventive purposes. They are sold in capsules because they are unpalatable in liquid form, and capsules are not suitable for young children. If your child's dry skin does not become lustrous with the diet I recommend and some flaxseed oil, a month-long trial of fish-oil supplementation will establish whether she needs omega-3 EFAs in the form in which they occur in fish.

Evening Primrose Oil and Black Currant Oil. Some children, like Jason, whose story I told earlier, need a higher intake of omega-6 EFAs than a balanced diet supplies. This is especially true of hyperactive children, those with allergies, and children who seem to be thirsty all the time. If your child's skin remains dry despite a healthy diet, flaxseed oil, and fish oils, then she may have an increased need for omega-6s.

One or two tablespoons of safflower oil a day may be useful, but a more efficient, and more expensive, source of omega-6s is evening primrose or black currant oil. This seed oil is unique in containing GLA, a fatty acid produced as an intermediate step during the metabolism of linoleic acid (LA). GLA enables a child's body to bypass the most common block in omega-6 metabolism.

The most reliable source of GLA is Efamol (brand) evening primrose oil. Its major commercial source in the United States is Murdoch Pharmaceuticals' Nature's Way line, found in health-food stores. Evening primrose oil comes in 500-milligram (mg) capsules, which can be swallowed by an older child or cut open so the oil can be rubbed on an infant's or small child's skin, through which it is slowly absorbed into her body. Dosage varies from one capsule a day for an infant to six capsules for an adolescent.

Since real primrose oil is expensive, a number of products claiming to offer GLA at a reduced price have appeared on the market. Some call themselves primrose oil, but in fact are mostly soy oil. Avoid them. Black currant oil has recently emerged as a source of GLA, too. One 250-milligram capsule is equivalent in GLA to one 500-milligram capsule of evening primrose oil. One brand of black currant oil is Eclectic Institute Inc., 11231 S.E. Market Street, Portland, Ore. 97216.

The FDA and Food Oils

Fish oils have proved effective in treating a large number of diseases in animal experiments and clinical trials with virtually no toxicity and a minimum of side effects. In humans, they help to lower cholesterol, triglycerides, and blood pressure; decrease complications of diabetes; improve arthritis, psoriasis, asthma, colitis, and migraines. In animals they help to prevent heart attacks, cancer, and autoimmune diseases. No drug or nutritional supplement has a comparable record of efficacy and safety in scientific studies. If you understand the widespread role of prostaglandins in disease and the effect of diet on prostaglandin formation, this record will not surprise you. Manufacturers of fish-oil concentrates have used this research to promote their products commercially, and the Food and Drug Administration has taken umbrage, asserting that such advertising makes fish-oil extracts drugs, not food supplements.

Evening primrose oil has shown more limited and inconsistent benefits in experimental and clinical studies, but some of its distributors have been even more vociferous in asserting its value in the treatment and prevention of illness. The FDA has recently imposed an import ban on primrose oil for that reason. Quarrels between the FDA and the companies that produce food oil capsules over what's a drug and what's a nutrient may make it difficult for you to obtain fish-oil or primrose oil capsules. This is a shame, but not a cause for alarm. Cod-liver oil is a suitable fish-oil source, and black currant seed oil is a suitable substitute for primrose oil.

In a more foolish and dangerous decision, the FDA has moved to limit the availability of flaxseed (linseed) oil to American consumers, claiming that its safety as a food oil has not been proved in this country. At the same time, there is *no restriction* on the use or sale of hydrogenated vegetable oils, even though numerous studies in animals show that the artificial fatty acids they contain may have toxic and undesirable effects. Hydrogenated oils have been in use for a mere fifty years, whereas flax oil has been a tradition in Northern and Central Europe for centuries and flax meal has been used for millennia. The safety of flax oil is documented and established by a long tradition of use. Alternatives to flax oil include cod-liver and walnut oils and unhydrogenated oils extracted from northern soy beans and winter wheat. The FDA's attempts to deny to American consumers access to flax oil is such a serious disservice to the people of this country that it warrants an investigation of the agency and the origins of that decision.

In the chapters that follow, I will outline for you how, during each stage of your child's life, from conception to young adulthood, you can help her build resistance to disease through an optimum intake of EFAs, their co-factor nutrients, and antioxidants, and by avoiding anti-nutrients. This book will resolve any confusion you have about the best diet for your child, and it will give you the advice you need to use nutritional supplements rationally and sensibly to give your child's body the extra boost it needs for maximum health. There is no magic here—just the foods and supplements that have been proved effective by research and in my own medical practice.

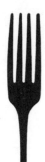

Pregnancy:
Optimally Nourished Mothers
Produce Stronger Babies

Your unborn child's future lies in your hands. From conception to birth, he will be completely dependent on you for the nourishment that will largely determine whether he is born healthy. A developing fetus gets all his nourishment from the placenta, which, in turn, is kept supplied by his mother's blood. So *everything* you take in—food, drinks, drugs, cigarette smoke—will affect your baby's development. What's more, he will depend on your immune system to protect him from germs that attack you. Since everything you ingest also affects the condition of your own body's defenses, it is very important for you to get enough minerals, vitamins, and EFAs, and to eat and drink as few anti-nutrients as possible.

The choices—what you eat, whether or not you smoke, whether you drink alcohol, what drugs you take—are all yours. If the child you are carrying is born with the healthiest possible body, he will have the foundation for a well-regulated defense system that will grow stronger as he grows older. Sure, you can start later in your child's life to counteract earlier nutritional mistakes, but why not start him off right?

The first three months of pregnancy are the most dangerous in terms of birth defects, because the cells of the embryo and fetus are multiplying and specializing very rapidly.

During the second and third trimesters, the embryo grows into a fully formed baby. This is when his immune cells develop, but they aren't yet able to do any work. Your own immune system does all the work for both of you. Not until three months after birth will your infant's immune system begin to protect him.

We know little about how the foods a mother eats specifically affect her unborn baby's immune system, but a great deal is known about the ways in which what you eat and drink affect his overall development. So it's a safe bet that good nutrition will help his immune system develop properly.

The first rule of good nutrition for a pregnant woman is one that will make food lovers happy: *Eat heartily.* Since your primary goal is to ensure good nutrition for your unborn baby, quantity, as well as quality, is important. *Do not skip meals, skimp on food, or attempt to diet during your pregnancy.*

This means that as long as you are eating nutritionally balanced meals, limiting the amount of weight you gain should never be a goal during pregnancy. If you start with a normal weight—not more than 20 pounds over what you should weigh for your height and bone structure—you must gain 25 to 35 pounds over nine months, simply to provide enough nourishment for your fetus to develop properly. Even if you are more than 20 pounds overweight at the beginning of your pregnancy, you must still gain from 24 to 27 pounds.

The weight you gain represents your baby, the placenta, the amniotic fluid, and your expanded breasts and blood volume. Any excess weight you carry before pregnancy is mainly fat, which will do your unborn baby little good. He will need protein, calcium, and all the other crucial minerals and vitamins. (If you are not sure whether your prepregnancy weight is normal, check the most recent Metropolitan Life height/weight tables. Many women feel they are overweight when their weight is normal, and normal only when they are quite thin. The tables should set you straight.)

What if you find you gain a lot of weight very quickly—if, say, in the first three to six months you put on all the weight you expected to gain over the entire nine-month period? The same advice still holds: Don't diet. It is far less dangerous to your baby's health for you to continue to gain weight. Once your baby is born, you can safely begin reducing your food intake. The larger your weight gain, the longer it takes to lose it. (But if you breast-feed, you will need to keep on eating for two until your baby is weaned.)

Are three meals a day enough? Probably not. During pregnancy, you will feel your best if you change your eating pattern to six small, low-fat, high-carbohydrate meals. Why? There are two reasons:

• Many minimeals will help keep you from overeating, because you will be less likely to want between-meal snacks.

• You may avoid three of the commonest conditions of pregnancy, *nausea, hypoglycemia,* and *hyperglycemia:*

Nausea. Also known as morning sickness, this is not an inevitable accompaniment to the earliest stages of pregnancy. When severe, it may actually be caused by nutritional deficiencies. A six-minimeal-a-day pattern will often relieve it. (For more information on nausea, see p. 46.)

Hypoglycemia. This is a condition in which blood sugar falls so low that not enough glucose gets to the brain; it is often the culprit when a pregnant woman faints. Hypoglycemia can also create hormonal swings that make you feel listless and down in the dumps. But, most crucial of all, *when your blood sugar is low, your developing infant's blood sugar is low, too—and lack of sufficient glucose can damage an unborn baby's brain.* So you want to avoid hypoglycemia.

Hyperglycemia. High blood sugar is technically the opposite of hypoglycemia. In fact, the two often accompany each other. The hormonal changes of pregnancy can produce wide swings in blood sugar with hyperglycemia being followed by hypoglycemia. Severe hyperglycemia is a sign of diabetes, a dangerous condition in pregnancy. A recent study from Italy, published in the *New England Journal of Medicine,* found that even the mildest degrees of hyperglycemia in pregnancy, generally considered normal, are associated with an increased frequency of birth defects, toxemia, cesarean section, and abnormal birth weights.[1] The best way to produce a stable blood sugar level, which does not swing too high or too low, is to eat frequent small meals that are high in soluble fiber and/or protein and low in sugar.

WHAT'S GOOD TO EAT AND DRINK
DURING PREGNANCY
—AND WHAT TO AVOID

In the pages that follow, I will be giving you a lot of specific information about the foods and drinks that will help you create a healthy baby and keep your own immune system in top form. Before I get into details, though, it might not be a bad idea to look at a few basic principles that can guide you to sound nutrition during pregnancy:

- *Choose foods that are low in fat and sugar and/or high in fiber.* This is a good strategy at any time, but it is crucial during pregnancy. If you get many of your daily calories from sugar or the wrong kinds of fats, such as those in fried or greasy foods, then you're not getting the extra vitamins and minerals you must have to meet the needs of your developing fetus and to keep turning those EFAs into prostaglandins for your own immune system. You are also consuming anti-nutrients that block your body's metabolism of EFAs—so you're doing *double* damage to your immune system.

  Fiber will protect you from that bane of pregnant women, constipation.

- *Make sure you get enough calcium to fill both your own needs and the needs of your developing infant.* As your embryo develops into an infant, he needs plenty of calcium to build sound bones and teeth. At the same time, your own body needs about 800 milligrams of calcium a day (the equivalent of three glasses of milk) to maintain your own bones and teeth. So you will need to consume much more calcium than usual. If you don't add enough calcium to your diet, your baby will take what he needs from *your* teeth and bones.

- *Be wary of prepared, packaged, and frozen foods; vitamin pills and mineral supplements; and all drugs: read labels carefully.* As we saw in Chapter 1, manufactured foods generally contain generous amounts of such anti-nutrients as partially hydrogenated vegetable oils, salt, and sugar, so they re-

ally don't fit in with the principle of a low-fat, low-sugar
diet. Manufactured foods also contain very little in the way
of EFAs.

Vitamin pills and mineral supplements have to be approached
with caution because, as we shall discover in a few pages, the
wrong combinations can do more harm than good. And, in general,
drugs that are perfectly safe at other times have the potential to
do damage to a developing fetus. Look for warnings on packages
and inserts.

YOUR PREGNANCY DIET

Dairy Products

If you are able to digest them, dairy products are the best
source of calcium for both you and your unborn baby. They are
generally terrific sources of protein as well, so when you eat dairy
products, you are getting two essential nutrients for the price of
one.

Of course, whole-milk dairy products are high in fat, so low-
fat versions are usually best.

• *I recommend four servings of dairy products, or the equivalent in high-calcium nondairy foods, every day of your pregnancy.*

One serving of dairy products is

8 ounces of low-fat yogurt, milk, or cottage cheese
1½ ounces of low-sodium hard cheese.

You can substitute twice as much (3 ounces) of soft white
goat cheese (chèvre) for hard cheese, but because other kinds of
soft cheeses, such as brie, generally contain more water, you
would have to eat twice as much to get as much calcium. And this
brings you up against the main problem of cheese—high fat content. Don't eat more than one serving of hard or goat cheese a
day. It is a good idea to avoid cream cheese altogether. It is
virtually pure fat, and has very little nutritional value.

If you follow this plan, you will get 1,100 milligrams of calcium each day from dairy products, plus a few hundred more from other foods. This is enough for your own and your baby's requirements, so you won't need to take a calcium supplement.

If you want to, you can double the calcium content of a single serving of yogurt, milk, or cottage cheese by mixing in ⅓ cup of nonfat dry milk powder. This adds 80 calories.

What if you have a lactose intolerance and can't digest dairy products? You can still get plenty of calcium from other foods. Here are five nondairy equivalents to one serving of milk:

> 4 ounces of canned fish with bones (fresh fish won't give you the same amount of calcium unless you eat the bones).
> ½ cup of (fresh) kale or collard greens.
> 5 corn tortillas (the calcium comes from lime used in their preparation).
> 2 cups of dried beans—red or kidney beans, white or fava beans, or chick-peas.
> ⅔ cup nuts. Almonds and filberts are highest in calcium. Walnuts and pecans are only fair. Peanuts don't count, since they aren't really nuts at all. Pistachios have little calcium.
> ⅔ cup seeds. Pumpkin seeds are excellent, sunflower fair to good.

Fish, Poultry, and Meat

The key here for meat is lean and low-fat.

• *You should eat at least 6 ounces of fish, poultry, or lean meat, or a vegetarian equivalent, every day of your pregnancy.*

Try to eat at least 12 ounces (three 4-ounce servings) of *fresh* oily, cold-water fish—salmon, tuna, mackerel, herring, sardines, or bluefish—every week. These fish are rich in omega-3 EFAs, which are vital for the developing nervous system of your fetus, and may also be important for his developing immune system.

Your own immune system will be working for two, so you need omega-3 EFAs to keep it running properly. Research has shown that during pregnancy a woman's immune system becomes slightly depressed, probably in order to keep her body from rejecting the developing embryo as if it were a parasite. It is all the more important, then, that you provide your immune system with as much nourishment as possible, so as not to weaken it any further!

Remember that fish vary in EFA content, and that processing and cooking can deplete or damage EFAs. White-fleshed fish such as sole or flounder contain few EFAs to start with. Fresh tuna, salmon, and bluefish are excellent grilled or poached, or eaten cold in salads. Anchovies, herring, and shrimp are nice additions to salads, also. (I don't recommend sushi or sashimi, which are increasingly popular in this country. Raw fish can contain parasites—always cook fish before you eat it.) Mackerel can be used in fish stews or soups. And one great American luxury seafood—lobster—is a fair source of EFAs, so indulge yourself.

What about canned tuna? It's a fair source, especially white albacore. But the oil used in the canning process is usually a vegetable oil low in omega-3s. Canning in water also lowers the EFA content, so canned fish is nutritionally inferior to fresh fish. If possible, broil, bake, or poach your fish and broil or roast your poultry and meat. If you want to stir-fry or sauté, use a small amount of olive oil. A tablespoon will do for a family's meal. I like olive oil better than vegetable oil for cooking because vegetable oils oxidize in heat to form harmful peroxides. Peroxides function like sparks to damage EFAs, not to mention your body's cells, and may contribute to cancer. Olive oil resists peroxidation.

Olive oil also smokes easily, which means that you have to cook at a relatively low temperature. This helps preserve such nutrients as B vitamins and vitamin C. Vitamin C, you will recall, is one of the essential vitamins that help your body turn EFAs into the prostaglandins that keep your immune system humming.

If you blanch some green leafy vegetable, such as spinach, in the pan first with a little water and some herbs, you can steam your fish or poultry—or even your meat—without fat in an ordinary frying pan. This method also has the advantage of requiring a relatively low heat.

You needn't deprive yourself of red meat. It has received a bad press lately because even lean red meat contains more fat, especially more saturated fat, than fish or poultry. But red meat is rich in iron and zinc—both of which are important in helping your body metabolize EFAs—and are crucial nutrients for your developing fetus. Dark meat poultry, also under a cloud because it is fattier than white meat, is actually more nutritious than white

meat. If you like it, go right ahead and eat it. During pregnancy, you need to be more concerned with supplying essential nutrients for both you and your developing fetus than with protecting yourself against future heart disease. The fat in meat goes along with the nutrients you need. The idea is to avoid *added* fat, which contains no other nutrients. So buy the leaner cuts of steak, such as round, and trim the fat off; trim the skin off your dark meat chicken and turkey, if you wish, and enjoy the meat.

What if you are a vegetarian, or simply want some alternatives to fish, poultry, or meat? There are many good nonmeat sources of protein. You can substitute eggs, beans, or nuts, using the following guidelines:

> For 1 ounce of meat:
> 1 egg
> ¼ cup of cooked dried beans
> For 3 ounces of meat:
> ½ cup of nuts or seeds

Beans provide particularly good food value because they supply several essential nutrients and health factors besides protein, among them, as we have seen, calcium. Magnesium and copper in beans help your body process EFAs into the right prostaglandins. The fiber in beans helps prevent constipation. *You should eat at least 2 cups of cooked beans a week.* If flatulence is a problem, try soaking the beans overnight, discarding the soak water, and rinsing. This removes complex sugars that are the cause of flatulence for many. Or use bean curd (tofu) rendered more digestible by its processing. By pressing any type of bean through a strainer you can create a bean purée that is free of the skin. You lose fiber by this process, but this will usually eliminate flatulence.

The protein value of beans is enhanced by combining them with whole grains. Any serious vegetarian must become familiar with Frances Moore Lappé's *Diet for a Small Planet* and its companion book, *Recipes for a Small Planet* by Ellen Buchman Ewald. Both focus on combining grains, seeds, nuts, beans, and dairy products for high-protein meatless menus. A weakness of these books, though, is their lack of attention to other nutrients.

Peanuts are not true nuts; they are legumes, like beans, and have a comparable protein value, although their fatty acid compo-

sition is inferior. Other seeds and nuts that are good sources of protein include sunflower, sesame, and pumpkin seeds, and cashews and black walnuts.

Vegetables

These are an important source of vitamins C and A, both crucial for your fetus's development and for your own immune system. Vitamin C is essential for prostaglandin production, while vitamin A helps your immune system produce the lymphocytes that identify and kill enemy invaders. While you are pregnant, your own lymphocytes are thinking for two, so you want to keep them healthy. Your own skin, eyes, and cells also need vitamin A.
• *You should eat four servings of vegetables every day of your pregnancy.*
The best vegetable sources for both C and A are tomatoes, broccoli, asparagus, kale, and peppers. Brussels sprouts and cauliflower are rich sources of vitamin C. Carrots, spinach, squash, and sweet potatoes are all excellent sources of vitamin A.
Vegetables are one of the most nutritious snack foods you can eat, and they contain almost no fat. Keep your refrigerator stocked with such vegetable crunchies as raw zucchini and carrot sticks, cauliflower florets, pepper slices, cherry tomatoes, and celery. Sweet, crisp, fresh snow peas make delicious snacks too, as do fresh young green beans.

Fruits

Oranges, grapefruit, and strawberries are rich in vitamin C, a helper vitamin for EFAs. Apples and berries are good sources of fiber.

Bread, Potatoes, Pasta, and Cereals

These complex-carbohydrate foods are important sources of fiber and B vitamins. Vitamin B-6 helps turn EFAs into prostaglandins, to keep your immune system in tune.
Complex carbohydrates also contain very little fat, except what is used to prepare them.
• *Eat four servings a day from this group of foods.*

One serving is the following:

1 slice of bread
½ cup of dry cereal
⅓ cup of cooked cereal
1 medium potato

Choose whole-grain breads and cereals (preferably those with no sugar added, such as whole wheat shredded wheat or homemade granola such as the one in the recipe section of Chapter 10), brown rice, barley, buckwheat groats (sold in supermarkets as kasha), whole wheat pasta, and our old friends dried beans. (This makes beans a four-star food, offering you protein, calcium, and magnesium, as well as all the virtues of a complex carbohydrate.)

Read the ingredients list on any box of dry cereal, not only for sugar content but also for partially hydrogenated vegetable oil, an arch anti-nutrient, and salt.

Eat potatoes baked, boiled, or roasted. Skip the French fries—they add unnecessary fat and they are a big source of anti-nutrient peroxides.

Spreads, Toppings, and Condiments

Sour cream is added fat—use plain low-fat yogurt instead.

Low-fat yogurt, seasoned with chives and garlic, makes a delicious spread for potatoes. Yogurt with dill or chives and/ or garlic also goes well with most vegetables, whether cooked or raw. My tofu-based spread (see Chapter 10) is also delicious on potatoes and vegetables. Stay away from margarine and imitation butter, both full of the partially hydrogenated vegetable oil that is so destructive to your immune system. Butter, a source of vitamin A, is actually much less a dietary villain than these two highly touted substitutes.

Nut butters—almond, peanut, sesame—make great spreads for bread. Although they are high in calories, they are rich in minerals and EFAs. Be sure to get the unsalted variety.

If you want mayonnaise, use my recipe in Chapter 10, or buy a brand that's made with unhydrogenated soy oil. Don't use more than a tablespoon a day of the ordinary kind. My tofu mayonnaise is so nutritious that you can use as much as you want.

As we saw in Chapter 1, you can mix flaxseed oil half and half with virgin olive oil as a base for salad dressing. Yogurt or soft tofu mixed with vinegar and herbs work well, too. (See recipes in Chapter 10.) *Many commercial salad dressings are poison to the immune system because they contain partially hydrogenated vegetable oil.*

Seasonings and Cooking Oils

Avoid table salt altogether.
- Your body only needs 2,000 milligrams of sodium a *day.* Pregnancy increases that to 3,000 milligrams. But it is estimated that the average American consumes *7,000 milligrams* of sodium every day, *over twice the daily requirement for a pregnant woman. The salt that is naturally contained in a balanced diet is all you need, even during pregnancy.*

Among other things, salt helps to expand the volume of blood needed to nourish your placenta. But salt also contributes to fluid retention and can elevate your blood pressure—both common complications in the last months of pregnancy.

Cook without salt or soy sauce—there are excellent cookbooks telling you how to prepare delicious meals without salt, using lemon, herbs, and spices instead. Don't add salt at the table.

Whenever possible, ask restaurants to prepare your order without salt. Never add salt at the restaurant table, either. Avoid soy sauces and most other commercial sauces because of their high salt content.

Be very wary of packaged and prepared foods. Even those that appear to be healthy may contain large amounts of sodium. A single can or package of soup may contain as much as 800 to 900 milligrams, almost a third of the salt a pregnant woman should consume in an entire day. Avoid canned foods, or at least look for canned vegetables and soups prepared without salt. *Always read labels carefully; the sodium content is listed on almost all prepared and packaged foods manufactured in this country.*

WHAT YOU SHOULD AND SHOULD NOT DRINK

In addition to milk, which is a food as well as a drink, you will want to drink plenty of water during your pregnancy.

• *Do not drink chlorinated tap water. Drink only bottled spring water or well water that has been checked for purity.*

City tap water is always chlorinated and may contain a variety of environmental pollutants. In addition, it may contain lead leached in from the soldering on pipe joints. A study at the University of Perugia in Italy points to the possibility that substances produced by chlorination can damage genes.[2] Leached-in lead can damage the fetus's developing brain, leading to retardation and other problems. And environmental pollutants are potent anti-nutrients. Well water should be tested for potability every few years, and if you have reason to doubt the purity of yours, arrange with a water-testing service to examine it for microbes that are not included in the usual potability test. Run the water for three minutes to clear the water that has been standing in the pipes before taking any for food or drink. A charcoal filter on the spigot is not effective against lead or chlorine, but can eliminate many chemical pollutants.

Bottled mineral waters are usually all right. Club soda and seltzer should be made from filtered spring water and should contain no added salt.

• *Avoid any drink containing caffeine or alcohol.*

Any pregnant woman concerned about having a healthy baby should avoid such caffeine-containing drinks as coffee, tea, cocoa, and chocolate milk, and soft drinks such as colas.

Pregnancy makes your body two-thirds less able to metabolize caffeine. *When you are pregnant, one cup of coffee is as potent as three.* So if you drink two cups, the effect is the same as six.

Alcohol can lower a baby's birth weight and has been linked with neurological damage and delayed development in infants. It is also a powerful anti-nutrient that prevents your immune system from getting the prostaglandins it needs. Remember that a glass of wine, a bottle of beer, and a shot of liquor all contain approximately the same amount of pure alcohol—½ ounce.

As for the new nonalcoholic beers and wines, most contain chemical additives whose effect is unknown.

• *The hard truth about soft drinks.* They can do nothing but harm to your developing fetus and to your own immune system. They contain sugar, an anti-nutrient, and no nutrients. No-cal soft drinks contain NutraSweet, or aspartame, which has been proven, in laboratory studies, to harm the brains of young animals. If you drink it (or eat it in low-cal desserts or in hot drinks as Equal), you can't be sure it won't do the same to your fetus.

What's more, studies suggest that one effect of aspartame may be to increase your own appetite for sugar-containing sweets—thus completely defeating their purpose and leading you to add more anti-nutrients to your diet.[3]

Many soft drinks also contain caffeine and phosphoric acid. Phosphoric acid blocks the absorption of calcium and magnesium by your intestines. This makes it an anti-nutrient that does harm to your immune system, because magnesium is the most important of the helper minerals that keeps prostaglandin production properly regulated. And prostaglandins, in turn, keep your immune system regulated.

ABOUT SMOKING

• *Don't smoke.* Smoking doubles your risk of bearing a baby with a low birth weight. According to the National Academy of Sciences, underweight infants are more prone to serious diseases and more likely to have congenital conditions such as cerebral palsy, mental retardation, seizures, and vision problems.

Harvard researchers have discovered that in babies whose mothers smoke, lung size is reduced by 10 percent—a factor, according to the *New England Journal of Medicine*, that may contribute to the higher rate of respiratory disease in the children of smokers. Recent research has also found that maternal smoking in pregnancy increases the risk of childhood cancer by 50 percent.[4] If you are a smoker, don't resume smoking after your pregnancy ends. Numerous studies have documented the hazards of passive smoking (breathing someone else's cigarette smoke). For children, the immediate risk is an increase in the frequency, severity, and chronicity of respiratory disease.[5]

CAN YOU TAKE DRUGS DURING PREGNANCY?

• *Not unless absolutely necessary, and not at all during the first three months.* As we saw earlier, the first three months are the most crucial in terms of birth defects. But your developing fetus is at risk during your entire pregnancy. So avoid drugs such as marijuana and cocaine, both of which have been linked to birth defects.

Stay away from such prescription and over-the-counter medical drugs as antihistamines, aspirin, Tylenol, and Advil; sleeping pills; and pain-killers such as Darvon.

Avoid antinausea medicines, if possible. Bendectin, a prescription drug used for over a decade to control nausea in pregnancy, was recently banned by the FDA because it is suspected of causing birth defects.

If you are prone to acne, beware of using Accutane, a prescription medication, both before your pregnancy and during the first three months. Women taking it have produced babies with marked abnormalities of the head and brain.

Read the label and the enclosed literature of every drug you consider taking while you are pregnant. Those considered dangerous will have a printed warning on the box and on an instruction sheet inside. But understand that drugs considered safe may not in fact *be* safe. Many warnings appear only after widespread side effects have been discovered.

THE QUESTION OF NUTRITIONAL SUPPLEMENTS

You will need to take some supplements while you are pregnant. Studies have shown that the addition of certain vital nutrients in the right amount (often well above current government recommendations) can help reduce the risk of birth defects and protect a pregnancy from complications. But beware of taking megadoses of any supplement. In many cases no one really knows what effect they will have on you or your unborn baby. What's more, when you take one vitamin or mineral you could be interfering with your own—or your unborn baby's—ability to use some other vital nutrient. This is especially true with minerals. The usual prenatal multivitamin-and-mineral pills ignore this important fact. Their use may actually *worsen* deficiencies of key minerals such as zinc, crucial for EFA metabolism, and manganese.[6]

For both these reasons, designing your own megadose program—even if you have taken megadoses before your pregnancy without apparent harm—is like performing a potentially dangerous experiment on your unborn baby.

In the pages that follow, I will provide a proven, sensible program of mineral and vitamin supplements that has been successfully followed by hundreds of my patients. I will also suggest specific supplements, and especially combinations of supplements, that you should avoid.

ESSENTIAL FATTY ACIDS

Most American women don't get enough omega-3 EFAs. One result is an epidemic of dry skin and hair, a bonanza for America's huge skin cream and hair-conditioner industries. Worse, though, as we saw in Chapter 1, EFA deficiency means an immune system that doesn't work as well as it should. Omega-3 EFAs are vitally important in regulating your own immune system and in helping your unborn baby's nervous system to develop properly. EFAs may also provide a special service in helping to prevent birth defects. And in animal studies, flaxseed oil, rich in both types of EFA, omega-6 and omega-3, has been shown to protect against cleft palate induced by a toxic drug.[7]

You *can* get enough EFAs—and the minerals and vitamins you need to help your body metabolize them and produce prostaglandins—from food alone, but it's not easy. What's more, there are no RDAs for EFAs yet, and you won't find them in most standard multivitamin formulas. In my experience, individual requirements for these crucial nutrients vary a lot, so you will want to keep yourself and your fetus well supplied.

- *I recommend a daily supplement of flaxseed oil or fish-oil extract.* One or two tablespoons of food-grade flaxseed oil (available at health-food stores and a few pharmacies or by writing to Omega Nutrition, 165–810 West Broadway, Vancouver, British Columbia V5ZYC9, or Allergy Resources, Box 2131, Port Washington, N.Y. 11050) can be taken as a "medicine," or used as salad oil. Don't use flaxseed oil for frying; heat plus air destroys its activity. If you prefer, you can take three 1-gram capsules of MaxEPA or Efamol Marine fish-oil extract instead.

MINERALS

Calcium

As I explained on pages 26–27, calcium is an essential nutrient for both you and your unborn baby. Without it, your fetus will not be able to develop sound bones and teeth, and if you don't provide extra amounts for him, he will take what he needs from your bones. Food is the best source of calcium, as it is for most nutrients; but many women can't digest dairy products and may not wish to eat beans, canned fish, nuts and seeds, or kale or collard greens every day. Enter the calcium supplement.

The tricky thing about calcium supplements is that they aren't always easily absorbed. Calcium carbonate, the cheapest form, comes from plain old chalk, oyster shells, or dolomite. Calcium carbonate is very alkaline, so stomach acid is essential to make it soluble for absorption. It should always be taken with meals, because that's when the stomach secretes more acid to digest food. But even then, many women don't produce enough stomach acid to absorb this form of calcium very well.

This makes calcium citrate a good choice for a supplement. It is made with calcium from chalk that is chemically compounded with citric acid, a chemical that occurs naturally in the body and helps supply energy. The result is so easily absorbed that any woman can take it, even without food.

Normally, your body carefully regulates the amount of calcium you absorb, so that if you take more than you and your unborn baby need, you will excrete the extra calcium in your feces. In a very few people, this regulation process doesn't work well, and those people are susceptible to kidney stones. But citrate makes calcium so soluble that, when taken with plenty of magnesium, it will not precipitate kidney stone formation even if you are prone to them.

- *If you are unable to eat the dairy or nondairy food sources of calcium outlined on pages 26–27 under* Dairy Products *you should take 750 to 1,000 milligrams of a calcium citrate supplement each day.* A good time to take calcium is at bedtime, so that you avoid blocking absorption of other key minerals (see list, p. 46). Also, blood calcium levels tend to fall overnight, so you help your bones more by taking calcium just before sleep.

In some people, calcium may cause constipation. This can be easily corrected by adding 100 to 200 milligrams of magnesium a day to the amounts recommended in the next section. The possibility of this minor annoyance is no reason to deprive your unborn baby of one of the most important nutrients you can give him.

Magnesium

This mineral is important both in its own right and as a balance to calcium intake. It is stored in your bones, where it helps them retain their calcium. If your magnesium supplies are low, you will lose more of the calcium you take in, making less available for you and your unborn baby. *For maximum effectiveness, most authorities recommend that you balance calcium and magnesium in a two-to-one ratio.* This means you should take one part of magnesium for every two parts of calcium. If you take 1,000 milligrams of calcium each day, or get that much in food, you should be getting 500 milligrams of magnesium. Some women, though, need twice as much magnesium or more—an amount equal to or greater than the amount of calcium they take in each day. If you are irritable, constipated, easily fatigued, have trouble sleeping, or get muscle cramps easily, you may have a magnesium deficiency.

Perhaps even more important, magnesium is an important nutrient in your unborn baby's development. A recent West German study of 1,000 pregnant women found that women who took magnesium supplements of 400 milligrams a day produced babies with higher birth weights and slightly higher Apgar scores. (This is a 10-point index of vitality and alertness given to babies immediately after birth.) Overall, these women also had fewer spontaneous abortions and suffered less from such complications of pregnancy as toxemia.[8]

Yet the RDA for magnesium is only 250 milligrams, raised to only about 350 milligrams for pregnant women. Many supplements, particularly multivitamins and mineral supplements, simply don't contain enough magnesium for a pregnant woman.

It's hard to get enough magnesium on a typical American diet, which is short on such magnesium-rich foods as beans and nuts. In addition, stress depletes the supplies of magnesium your bones and cells do contain. I frequently encounter magnesium deficiency, even in women who believe they are well nourished.

- *I recommend a magnesium supplement to all pregnant patients.* In addition to the amount you may be getting in food to balance your calcium intake, you will want to take from 300 to 400 milligrams each day to counter any possible deficiency. The amount depends on your weight:

100 lbs	300 mg
120 lbs	360 mg
140 lbs	420 mg
160 lbs	400 mg

If cramps, irritability, or insomnia persist, you should double the dosage. For a woman with normal kidney function, or for her unborn baby, the danger of overdosing on magnesium is practically nonexistent. At worst, too much may cause diarrhea, at which point you can reduce the supplement.

Should you take a supplement that combines calcium and magnesium? While such preparations are increasingly popular, most of them rely on calcium carbonate and magnesium oxide, a combination that may be difficult for your body to absorb. Magnesium oxide, like calcium carbonate, dissolves only in stomach acid—and, as we saw above, many women don't produce enough stomach acid to do the job. But there is another hitch, as well—the calcium carbonate may block absorption of the magnesium oxide.

In any case, calcium-magnesium tablets are often so tightly compacted that they pass intact right through your digestive system.

- *I recommend taking calcium and magnesium separately: calcium in the form of calcium citrate, and magnesium as magnesium citrate or magnesium chloride.*

There are a number of other minerals you should take as supplements in order to ensure that you are getting adequate amounts.

Iron

This is needed by your unborn baby in the development of her brain and to build her blood cells, including the crucial white blood cells of her immune system. If you don't supply extra iron for her, she'll take what she needs from supplies your own body needs. And it's very hard to get enough of this essential mineral to meet the needs of pregnancy from your food alone. That's why most prenatal vitamin supplements contain 20 milligrams of iron a day.

Zinc

This element is absolutely crucial in the development of your baby's thymus, the most important organ in the immune system. The thymus is a gland in which the T-cells, the brains of her immune system, will be produced and trained to do their job properly. Zinc also stimulates growth. And, like iron and calcium, if you don't supply extra amounts, your growing fetus will take what she needs from your own body's essential stores.

As we shall see on pages 43, 45, 46, your body's ability to use zinc is affected by other vitamins and minerals. A recent British study showed that the usual prenatal multivitamin supplements actually cause a 30 percent *reduction* in the amount of zinc a pregnant woman is able to absorb.[9]

Copper

Another mineral that is needed by your fetus for the proper development of her immune system and brain. Yet even nonpregnant women usually get much less copper than the RDA, which is 1.6 milligrams. A study done at Virginia Polytechnic Institute found that pregnant women eating food of their own choice are actually in negative copper balance (they use more copper than they consume); their zinc and copper status was improved significantly by supplementation.[10]

• *High-EFA foods—beans, nuts, seafood, and the organ meats liver and kidney—are also good sources of iron, zinc, and copper.*

Manganese

Needed to help prevent birth defects,[11] it is found in whole grains and nuts, but the iron supplements you must take during pregnancy will block its absorption.

Trace Elements

These are minerals your body needs in amounts less than 1 milligram a day. *Selenium* helps prevent birth defects, cancer, and heart disease. *Chromium* helps your body's insulin keep your blood sugar stabilized, an important job during pregnancy because hyperglycemia and hypoglycemia can harm your baby (see p. 24). You donate a lot of chromium to your baby during pregnancy, and with each succeeding pregnancy your chromium depletion increases. *Iodine* is essential for the development of your unborn baby's thyroid gland. Iodine deficiency during pregnancy produces a mentally retarded baby. Luckily, seafood is a rich source of iodine. *If you don't eat three servings of seafood a week, you need an iodine supplement.*

VITAMINS

A strong argument for taking vitamin supplements during pregnancy is provided by studies that link vitamin deficiencies to birth defects. And you *can* have a vitamin deficiency even if you are getting the RDA, which may not be large enough to protect you and your developing baby during your pregnancy. This is particularly true of the B vitamins. Several studies have shown that multivitamin supplements taken throughout pregnancy could be an important step in preventing such birth defects as *spina bifida,* in which the spinal vertebrae are incompletely formed; other spinal defects; and cleft palate.[12]

One B vitamin, *vitamin B-6,* is important in helping EFAs make the prostaglandins that regulate your immune system. It is marginally deficient in 50 percent of pregnant women.[13] The current RDA for B-6 is 2 milligrams a day, yet a recent study at the University of Florida showed that a dose of 20 milligrams or more, over *ten times* the RDA, may be needed just to maintain normal blood levels during pregnancy. And according to the same study, 10 to 20 milligrams of B-6 a day produced newborns with 10 percent higher Apgar scores than those attained by babies whose mothers took less than 10 milligrams a day.[14]

An added benefit of B-6 is that it may help prevent hand pain, a surprisingly common problem in pregnancy. *The Journal of the Canadian Medical Association* reports that up to 25 percent of pregnant women suffer from *carpal tunnel syndrome:* pain and tingling in the palms and fingers and weakness in the thumbs. Several other studies, including one at the University of Washington, have linked this syndrome with B-6 deficiency. Women with carpal tunnel syndrome may need 100 to 500 milligrams a day to correct their deficiency.[15]

Haven't there been reports that vitamin B-6 is toxic in high doses? True—a report in the *New England Journal of Medicine* told of a few people who developed reversible nerve damage after consuming exceptionally high doses of vitamin B-6 —2,000 milligrams or more a day—for several months. At this megadose level, it appears that vitamin B-6 can actually block its own effect in the body. The doses I usually recommend to pregnant women—25 milligrams a day (10 to 25 times the RDA)—are, however, absolutely nontoxic. On the contrary, most women need this amount to help counteract environmental pollutants such as herbicides, which interfere with the body's ability to use B-6.

Folic acid, part of the B-complex of vitamins, helps your body turn out white blood cells, without which your immune system has no army with which to fight germs. What's more, folic acid deficiency causes anemia. Your body's folic acid requirements double during pregnancy, and in my experience folic acid deficiencies are very common in pregnant women who don't take supplements.

Vitamins A and C are essential co-factor vitamins in the metabolism of EFAs, so you need good supplies to keep your immune system well regulated.

High doses of vitamin C don't appear to do any harm to a developing baby (contrary to one report, they will not produce a baby so conditioned to high levels of vitamin C that he gets scurvy without them). But too much vitamin A can cause birth defects.

If you're even *thinking* about getting pregnant, don't take over 10,000 IU (international units) a day.

Vitamin E in doses of 200 IU per day (about 5 times the RDA) appears to be useful in preventing spontaneous abortion ("miscarriage").[16] Choline, sometimes classified as a B vitamin, should not be taken in pregnancy, nor should lecithin supplements, which are a common source of choline. Studies with pregnant rats show that maternal use of lecithin affects the developing brain cells of the fetus, producing abnormal behavior in the offspring.[17] The reason is probably related to the body's use of choline in making a *neurotransmitter* (nerve chemical) called acetylcholine. Higher than normal levels of such neurotransmitters in the fetal brain may cause permanent neurological changes. It is likely that other natural substances used by the body to make other neurotransmitters may also be toxic to the developing brain. These would consist primarily of individual amino acids, such as tryptophan, tyrosine, phenylalanine, and glutamine, which are used to control appetite, mood, pain, and insomnia. The toxic effect of aspartame (NutraSweet) on very young animals probably shares a similar mechanism, because NutraSweet consists of the amino acids phenylalanine and glutamic acid.

HOW YOU SHOULD TAKE YOUR VITAMINS AND MINERALS

Can you take minerals and vitamins in multimineral and multivitamin supplements, or even in a single multivitamin-and-mineral tablet or capsule? This is the form in which many people are accustomed to getting their minerals and vitamins. They are widely sold and are appealing because they seem to simplify the whole process of taking supplements. But, as with calcium and magnesium, there are many combinations of minerals, and of vitamins and minerals, that should not be taken at the same time. Calcium can block the body's ability to absorb zinc, iron, and copper. Zinc interferes with the absorption of iron, and vice versa. High doses of vitamin C and / or zinc will block absorption of selenium. And too much zinc can deplete the body's copper and manganese levels. The combination of B-1, B-12, vitamin C, and copper may produce a substance known as a vitamin B-12 analogue—a chemical similar to B-12 but which in fact blocks the action of B-12 in the body.[18] Both you and your developing fetus need B-12 to make blood cells—including those all-important immune-system white blood cells—and to help your brains and nerves work properly.

And because the RDAs of most vitamins don't account for your body's special needs during pregnancy, many of the most popular multivitamin and mineral supplements, including the most-prescribed prenatal supplements, simply do not provide high enough doses to be effective.

What's more, some supplements contain undesirable elements. Bioflavonoids are popular these days, and are included in some vitamin C supplements. Unfortunately, the bioflavonoid rutin can be converted in the intestine into another bioflavonoid, quercetin, that can damage chromosomes—leading to potential genetic damage in a developing fetus.[19] You'd be smart to avoid bioflavonoids during pregnancy, especially during the critical first three months.

• *During pregnancy, I recommend taking each vitamin and mineral separately, and in combinations that will not interfere with absorption or use by the body.*

The following lists provide a simple, safe, effective program of dosages, with a schedule that will allow maximum effectiveness for each supplement. (You will take most supplements with meals to give your body the best chance to absorb them.)

WHAT SUPPLEMENTS TO TAKE EACH DAY DURING YOUR PREGNANCY

ESSENTIAL FATTY ACIDS

As a liquid: 1 to 2 tablespoons of food-grade flaxseed oil per day. To maximize absorption, take right before or after a meal. Or use in dressings on salads, vegetables, and pasta. *Do not fry with it; high heat and air destroy EFAs.* You may substitute 1 teaspoon to 1 tablespoon of cod-liver oil.

In capsules: Three to six 1-gram capsules of fish-oil extract per day. (It will require 15 to 30 flaxseed oil capsules a day to equal 1 to 2 tablespoons of flaxseed oil.) Max-EPA or Efamol Marine are standard brands.

VITAMINS SUMMARIZED

VITAMIN	DAILY DOSAGE
A	10,000 units, or 1 tablespoon cod-liver oil, or one 8-ounce glass carrot juice (best choice)
B Complex	
B-1	10 mg
B-2	10 mg
B-3	100 mg
B-6	20–30 mg
B-12	10–20 micrograms (mcg)
Folic acid	800 mcg
Pantothenic acid	200 mg
Biotin	300 mcg
C	1,000 mg
D	400 units, or 1 teaspoon cod-liver oil
E	400 units, as d-Alpha-tocopherol (its most active form)

MINERALS SUMMARIZED

MINERAL	DAILY DOSAGE
Calcium	750–1,000 mg (calcium citrate)
Magnesium	300–600 mg (magnesium citrate or magnesium chloride)
Iron	30–60 mg, with food and vitamin C
Zinc	15–20 mg The best form is zinc citrate or zinc picolinate. Do *not* take with iron.
Manganese	5 mg Do *not* take with iron.
Copper	2 mg, with vitamin C.
Selenium	200 mcg The best form is selenomethionine. Do *not* take with zinc or vitamin C.
Chromium	400 mcg Take the GTF (glucose-tolerance factor) form because, bound to an organic complex, the chromium is easily absorbed.
Iodine	200 mcg *only* if you *do not* eat seafood

WHEN TO TAKE WHAT

*The following list will enable you to get the most value
from your supplements.*

MEAL		EFA SOURCE
Breakfast	*Vitamins*	A
		B-1
		B-2
		B-3
		B-6
		Folic acid
		Pantothenic acid
		Biotin
		C
		D
	Minerals	Iron
		Copper
Lunch	*Vitamin*	E
	Minerals	Magnesium
		Selenium
		Chromium
		Iodine
Supper	*Vitamin*	B-12
	Minerals	Zinc
		Manganese
Bedtime	*Mineral*	Calcium citrate

HOW FOOD AND SUPPLEMENTS CAN OVERCOME MORNING SICKNESS

Eat for nausea? That sounds like a contradiction, and no one is exactly sure why it works, but it often does. Time and time again, I have found that my patients have been able to stop morning sickness by doing exactly what they had been avoiding—eating, and eating well.

Eat small meals of low-fat foods. Fats will make your nausea worse. Whole wheat bread or oatmeal, salt-free crackers, rice, fish, and vegetables are good choices. Meat, nuts, fruit, and dairy products may contribute to your nausea.

If food alone doesn't clear up the nausea, and the problem is severe enough to limit weight gain, I turn to supplements, which nearly always work. My own theory is that poor nutrition and hormonal changes produce deficiencies of vitamin B-6 and vitamin K, which interfere with the activity of key enzymes that regulate the function of the nausea center in the brain. Patients I have been treating nutritionally before their pregnancies uniformly report less nausea than in earlier pregnancies. If I don't see a patient until she's already pregnant, urgent measures may be needed.

When Linda came to me during her pregnancy because she was nauseated and vomiting frequently, I gave her an initial dose of 100 milligrams of vitamin B-6, followed by an injection of 10 milligrams of vitamin K. She went home and, under my orders, continued taking 100 milligrams of B-6 a day for a week. By the end of the week, Linda's nausea had cleared up. The rest of her pregnancy was normal.

- *For morning sickness, I recommend 100 to 200 milligrams of B-6 and 10 milligrams of vitamin K a day.* Occasionally, more than 200 milligrams a day is necessary, but this amount should only be taken under a physician's supervision. I also give patients an initial injection of vitamin K, which works in a day or two. Taken orally, the Vitamin K takes somewhat longer to produce results—about ten days.

HOW MUCH SHOULD YOU EXERCISE DURING PREGNANCY?

It is fashionable today for young mothers to start or continue with a program of strenuous aerobic exercise during pregnancy. *Exercise is beneficial, but I think there is a danger in strenuous exercise during pregnancy.*

In animal studies, internal temperatures in the range of 102° F. increase the frequency of birth defects. Strenuous aerobic exercise, especially distance running, can easily raise body temperature to that level, imperiling your health and that of your unborn child. If you are already an experienced runner, plan to keep your distances under 6 miles a day during pregnancy. If you have not been active before, your best bets for exercise are swimming, stationary cycling, or brisk walking. Start with short times or distances, and always warm up before you start. (A brisk walk is good, as are leg-lifts, and "bicycling" with your legs in the air while lying on your back. These last two exercises strengthen your abdominal muscles and your legs as well as warming you up.)

If you feel comfortable, you can exercise right through pregnancy. But remember—don't try to set any records. Exercise only as long as it feels comfortable. Anyone with a medical history of miscarriages should consult a physician before beginning any exercise program.

LEARN TO RELAX SO YOUR BODY CAN DO ITS JOB

When you're pregnant, your body is working full time to create another human being. Adding to this the challenges and demands of a home, a career, and the nurture of other children, if you have them, can be very taxing to mind and body.

Stress, whether physical or emotional, can do harm during pregnancy. The increased adrenaline secreted during psychological stress can decrease the flow of blood to your fetus, particularly if stress is prolonged. In experiments, stressed animals have delivered litters of lower-than-average birth weight.

Make a conscious effort to take time out for yourself and to counter stress with calming meditation and relaxation exercises. Here are brief but effective breathing and relaxation exercises my patients use.

BREATHING EXERCISE

1. Stand with your arms at your sides.

2. Breathe out as much as you can through your nose.

3. To force more air out, contract your abdominal muscles strongly.

4. Breathe in slowly through both nostrils.

5. Fill the lower part of your lungs by letting your abdominal muscles relax so your abdomen bulges out.

6. Keep breathing in and fill the middle part of your lungs by expanding your rib cage.

7. Finish breathing in and fill the upper part of your lungs by raising your shoulders.

8. Breathe out slowly.

9. Let your rib cage contract.

10. Finally, tighten your diaphragm and abdominal muscles to empty your lungs of air.

Repeat three times.

RELAXATION EXERCISE

The purpose of this exercise is to stretch muscles that most people keep chronically tense. This promotes relaxation.

1. Follow Breathing Exercise.

2. Sit comfortably in a chair that supports your arms. Notice how much tension is present in your shoulders. Pull your shoulders down toward your hips, feeling their movement. Let them return to a neutral position and feel how much more relaxed they are. Let this feeling of relaxation travel from your shoulders down both arms into your hands.

3. Open your hands as wide as you can. Stretch your fingers. Feel each finger pulling away from every other finger and from the center of your palm. Do this for five seconds and then stop, relax, and let your hands assume a natural position. Feel how relaxed they are.

4. Now pay attention to your legs, from your feet up to your hips. Feel how much tension is in them. Stretch your legs out, raising your heels 3 or 4 inches from the floor. Begin the stretch in your heels and pull through your knees to your hips. Point your toes gently toward your face. Feel the stretch in your legs and then let them relax. Feel how relaxed they are. Let the relaxation spread up your thighs and into your lower back.

5. Pay attention to your jaws. Feel how tense they are. Keeping your mouth closed, push your chin down toward your chest. Let your tongue hang naturally in the middle of your mouth; don't push it down, or up to the roof of your mouth. Feel the muscles in your cheeks stretching. Now relax your jaws. Feel how relaxed they are.

6. Turn your attention to your forehead and eyes. Close your eyes gently, just letting your lids drop. Imagine a hand caressing your forehead, starting at your eyebrows and caressing upward, smoothing all the wrinkles and continuing over the top of your head, down the back of your neck, and into your shoulders.

7. Now repeat steps 2 through 6.

Note: Natural childbirth classes often include relaxation exercises, and these can be used when you feel tense. But the breathing exercises you learn in natural childbirth classes are intended for use during labor; they won't help calm you during pregnancy.

THE LAST WORD: SLEEP

Pregnant women need the health-promoting rest of a good night's sleep. But sleeping pills may cause birth defects, and tryptophan, otherwise a safe, nonchemical sleep aid, can be carcinogenic in a pregnant woman's body. Why? Because your body maintains a high estrogen level during pregnancy, and estrogen acts to convert tryptophan into a carcinogen.

- *Take calcium citrate and/or magnesium citrate or chloride.* Calcium and magnesium encourage sleep. If your bedtime calcium supplement doesn't help you sleep, try taking magnesium at bedtime. If you don't use a calcium supplement because you get all the calcium you need from food, take just the magnesium at bedtime. Keep raising the magnesium dose until you get diarrhea or a good night's sleep.

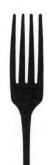

From Birth to Six Months— Creating High Health: Should You Breast-Feed?

Should a busy working mother take the time and trouble to breast-feed her infant? Despite the convenience of bottles and formulas, modern research has shown that the answer is a resounding *yes!* Studies show that bottle-fed infants get sick more often than those who are breast-fed, because a newborn infant's immune system is not yet able to perform at peak levels. Breast milk contains substances that will protect her against allergies and many of the infections common to bottle-fed babies. Other substances help her immune system to develop. What's more, recent evidence suggests that breast-feeding may produce straighter teeth than bottle feeding. And, as a dividend, breast-feeding offers some decided benefits to the new mother. It helps her recover more quickly from childbirth, it may protect her from breast cancer later in life, and it offers her some protection against conceiving again.

For the first six months of an infant's life, breast milk is the optimum food. For that reason, *I recommend that a new mother breast-feed as much as possible during her baby's first six months of life. Full-time breast-feeding is best, but part-time breast-feeding is the next-best thing you can do.* There are a few exceptions, which I shall discuss later (p. 61).

Breast-feeding while holding down a full-time job is difficult—it demands planning, flexibility, and the sympathetic cooperation of a care giver. To breast-feed full time, you will also need the right conditions at work. But the benefits for your new baby are so substantial that I urge you to consider attempting it anyway.

For a variety of reasons, some women are unable to breast-feed at all. If you have this problem, you can still protect your baby to some extent. Although no formula available today can provide the same protection as breast milk, it is possible to make up for some of the deficiencies of formulas with supplements, especially after the first three months.

In the pages that follow, I will show you what breast-feeding can do for your baby and for you. I will also outline complete feeding programs to provide the best possible nutrition for your newborn baby, whether you are able to breast-feed full time, part time, or not at all.

WHAT BREAST MILK CAN DO FOR YOUR BABY

A DIRECT BOOST TO HER IMMUNE SYSTEM

An infant's immune system is immature. It starts functioning as soon as she is born, but its lymphocytes are naïve—they have not yet met any of the thousands of different germs, bacteria, fungi, and other invaders they will encounter in her lifetime. They can respond to foreign bodies, but because they must start from scratch for each one, they are slow.

A newborn infant's lymphocytes are also not yet capable of making all the different kinds of antibodies she needs. They acquire that ability slowly over her first year of life. The last one they begin to make is the *IgA antibody,* which performs a crucial service: coating her intestinal and respiratory tracts, thus protecting them against infection. Because their bodies can't yet make the IgA antibody, infants under a year are particularly prone to intestinal-tract infections.

Fortunately, a newborn infant still has her mother's antibodies in her blood. They will augment her defenses during her first three months. After that, they are gone, but by that time her immune system has had a taste of the outside world and can handle some defensive jobs on its own. But because she still can't make that key IgA molecule, her intestinal tract remains vulnerable. Some of the special substances in breast milk are uniquely designed to protect your infant's intestinal tract from infection until she is ready to do it herself. Others enhance her overall defenses, while still others help her immune system strengthen and mature.

Let's take a look at these substances.

Bifidus Growth Factor. Bifidus is a lactobacillus, a good bacteria that guards against intestinal infection. It turns lactose, or milk sugar, into lactic acid, and lactic acid in turn discourages the growth of yeast, harmful bacteria, and parasites in the intestinal tract. Because of a growth factor in breast milk, bifidus thrives in the intestines of breast-fed babies. But because cow's milk contains no such factor, bifidus does not grow in the intestines of bottle-fed babies.

As an older infant's IgA levels rise, she doesn't need bifidus as much. When she starts to eat solid food, bifidus gradually disappears from her intestinal tract.

Immunoglobins. These are antibodies that protect your infant against a wide range of infections, particularly in her intestinal tract. They help make up for her inability to produce IgA antibodies.

Interferon. Genetically engineered interferon is being used experimentally against cancer and other diseases. Your body makes small amounts of it naturally, and it is contained in breast milk. It combats viruses that can cause intestinal infections, preventing them from replicating and spreading the infection.

Enzymes. Human milk (and only human milk) contains an enzyme that breaks down the fat in the milk to form individual, free fatty acids. These free fatty acids (both essential and nonessential) inhibit the growth of parasites in the intestine. They are especially effective at killing off *Giardia lamblia,* a one-celled parasite that is a common—and often unrecognized—cause of diarrhea in infants. *Giardia* infections are rampant in the United States, especially in mountainous areas. Beavers are an important reservoir of *Giardia* infection; they contaminate otherwise pure mountain streams. In cities, important sources of *Giardia* exposure are domestic pets and food handlers in restaurants. Breast-fed infants are more resistant to *Giardia* infection than those who are bottle fed. Heating, by the way, rapidly destroys this important enzyme.

Iron and Lactoferrin. Most infant formulas contain iron, up to two to three times more than breast milk. But the iron in formulas is not easily absorbed by a very young infant, and intestinal bacteria thrive on the unabsorbed iron in her digestive tract. This is where lactoferrin comes in. It is a protein that, in breast milk, combines with iron to make it more easily absorbed by an infant. What's more, lactoferrin inhibits the growth of bacteria to give your baby double protection.

Between three and six months of age, an infant becomes more able to absorb iron. From six to ten months, she may need extra iron if she is exclusively breast-fed, because breast milk may not contain enough. By this time, as her maturing immune system begins to produce IgA antibodies, she will be able to defend herself against bacterial infections in her intestines.

Zinc. Infant formulas are usually fortified with zinc, too, but, as with iron, the zinc in breast milk is more easily absorbed by an infant. Zinc is essential for the development of the thymus gland, in which T-cells are "educated" for their key role as the "mind" of the immune system: recognizing invaders and calling out the troops to do battle.

Antioxidants. In Chapter 1 we described the crucial role of the "antioxidant defense system" in protecting white blood cells when they burn germs. At such times, the white blood cells become tiny furnaces. They need antioxidant protection in order not to burn themselves up. And germ-burning white blood cells also give off free radicals, the "sparks" that can damage cell membranes, chromosomes, and enzymes. Antioxidants quench those sparks.

Selenium and Taurine. These are two key antioxidants contained in breast milk not added in sufficient amount to formulas. Breast milk contains three times more *selenium* than formulas. Studies have shown that when infants are breast-fed for two to three months and then switched to formula, the levels of selenium in their blood go down.[1] But infants who are breast-fed even part time for up to a year keep high levels of selenium in their blood. The selenium content of human milk, moreover, is influenced by the mother's own selenium levels.[2]

By the time they are a year old, bottle-fed infants begin to get selenium in their solid food. But from three to nine months, they suffer a temporary deficiency that can have dramatic consequences. Selenium-deficient animals are susceptible to infection because their white blood cells simply don't survive as well without antioxidant protection. Among humans, breast-fed infants hardly ever get chronic diarrhea, whereas bottle-fed infants frequently do. The ratio is a hundred to one. For every breast-fed baby who gets chronic diarrhea, one hundred bottle-fed babies get it.

In addition to its role as an antioxidant, *taurine* plays a critical role in brain development and digestion. Your body manufactures it from dietary protein, but your infant's body isn't able to do that yet. Taurine is not found in cow, soy, or goat's milk, and has only recently begun to be added to formulas.

Antioxidants such as selenium and taurine are probably important in preventing respiratory-tract infections, too, but these have not yet been studied as thoroughly as digestive-tract infections. The combined surface area of both systems—one of which filters all the air your child breathes, while the other filters all her food—is enormous. An adult's intestinal tract alone contains a surface the size of a tennis court. White blood cells protect this huge surface area against the infections to which it is continuously exposed—and antioxidants protect the white blood cells.

GLA. In Chapter 1, we found out how the body converts EFAs into prostaglandins, chemicals that in turn regulate the activity of the cells in the immune system. Prostaglandins are especially important to the health of lymphocytes. Enzymes in your liver convert the key omega-6 EFA, linoleic acid, or LA, into GLA, an important intermediate step on the road to prostaglandin production. But the immature livers of newborns and infants don't produce enough of the key enzyme to be able to make this conversion. As a result, bottle-fed infants are more prone to allergies. Breast-feeding bypasses the whole problem by supplying GLA directly to your infant.

ANTIALLERGY PROTECTION

Because breast milk contains GLA and other EFAs, breast-feeding can actually delay the onset of food allergies as well as other allergic symptoms such as rashes and nasal discharges.[3]

On the other hand, cow's milk in the first year, or too early feeding of solid food, will precipitate allergies. Why? Because an infant's intestinal tract is porous; it can't screen out the big molecules that cause allergies. This is why infants under a year old are particularly susceptible to food allergies, and why you should not feed an infant wheat, cow's milk, fish, or egg whites during her first year of life. It takes six to twelve months for an infant's intestinal tract to develop the ability to screen out allergenic molecules.

Jonathan's mother brought him to me when he was two. His family was very allergy-prone: both his parents had hay fever and asthma, and his older brothers each had multiple allergies. One had eczema. Jonathan's mother had breast-fed him for a whole year, and during that time he had not had a single allergy. But when he began to eat solid food, he, too, developed allergic symptoms, in the form of nasal congestion and eczema. Even so, his symptoms were much milder than those of his brothers, who had been bottle fed.

Jonathan might have avoided allergies altogether if his mother had been better nourished. She was very prone to colds, and her hair was dull and limp. All this, with the number and severity of her own allergic symptoms, suggested an EFA deficiency that had undoubtedly affected the quality of her breast milk, making it less protective for Jon than it might otherwise have been.

To give Jonathan's mother EFA protection, I started her on 1 tablespoon of flaxseed oil and 1 teaspoon of cod-liver oil daily. After six weeks, her hair became glossy and lustrous; that winter she went without a cold, and, as I expected, had fewer allergic symptoms.

For Jonathan, I prescribed 200 milligrams of vitamin C, 1 teaspoon of flaxseed oil, and 1 teaspoon of cod-liver oil, all given at once in his orange juice each day. After four weeks, he was no longer congested and sniffling, and his skin had become smooth to the touch. He looked shinier, happier, and more alive.

A breast-feeding mother, then, needs to keep herself well nourished, particularly in terms of EFAs. If you have a family history of allergies, I would suggest:
• *Breast-feed until your child weans herself.*

Delay the introduction of infant formula as long as you can; try for six months.

Ongoing research at Harvard Medical School and Boston Children's Hospital suggests that giving formula at too early an age to allergy-prone infants who are also being breast-fed can increase the risk of intestinal inflammation. The immune-stimulating effect of mother's milk makes the *very young* infant more likely to mount a strong immune response to any foreign protein that enters his intestine, whether the protein comes from an invading bacteria or from food. Dr. W. Allan Walker, an immunologist who heads the Combined Program in Pediatric Gastroenterology and Nutrition at Harvard, advises mothers not to mix breast and formula feeding if there is a history of milk allergy in their parents or siblings. If a mixed feeding program is necessary, Walker suggests the use of a hydrolyzed infant formula (such as Neutramigen) that is predigested and less allergenic.

Whether Walker's warnings apply to the first few weeks of life or the first few months is not known, and the final outcome of his research is still pending. As it now stands, this research is another piece of evidence against the use of formula feedings in the first few months of life.
• *Be sure that you are getting plenty of EFAs, especially the omega-3s.*
• *Start giving your baby flaxseed or walnut or cod-liver oil at six months.* (See p. 67 for tips on giving flaxseed oil to babies.) This last is good advice for any mother, whether or not her child is susceptible to allergies.

WHAT BREAST-FEEDING CAN DO FOR YOU

Breast-feeding is a terrific way to tighten the bond between you and your newborn because it calls for the kind of holding and touching that helps sensitize you to each other. As you watch your baby breast-feed, you are going to make eye contact with him—an important part of the growing closeness between the two of you. All this can be done fairly well with a bottle, although women who breast-feed often report intense internal sensations that can make them even more responsive to their infants.

A bottle can't help your body recover more quickly from childbirth. Nursing triggers the secretion of *vasopressin*, a hormone that makes the uterus contract, helping it return to its normal state more quickly than it would otherwise.

Breast-feeding may also protect you against developing breast cancer later in life. Scientists at the Fred Hutchinson Cancer Research Center in Seattle, Washington, report that women who breast-feed have half the risk of developing breast cancer compared with those who don't. The reason is not known yet, but the protection is clearly there.

As long as you breast-feed, you will be somewhat less fertile than usual—although, unfortunately, you can't really rely on this factor as a contraceptive. Breast-feeding elevates your body's levels of *prolactin*, a hormone that tends to inhibit ovulation—but not 100 percent! (One contraceptive method *not* to use is an IUD. We now know that the risk of perforating your uterus with an IUD inserted while breast-feeding is about ten times that for one inserted after the infant is weaned.)

As a final bonus, full-time breast-feeding burns about 250 calories a day, the equivalent of a 3-mile run. This can help offset the fact that you will still be eating more than you normally would. You can cut the amounts of food you ate while you were pregnant by 25 percent (from 2,500 calories a day to about 1,900). As a result, while you are breast-feeding you should begin to lose about half a pound a week.

Although you may be eager to lose more than 2 pounds a month, I don't recommend it. A strict diet may jeopardize the quality of your breast milk, with potential repercussions for your baby's health. In a University of Utah study, researchers observed twelve women who breast-fed for ten weeks after giving birth. On a 1,500-calorie-a-day diet, all the women complained of fatigue and said their babies didn't seem satisfied with their feedings. In addition, all the mothers produced fewer than the 22 to 24 ounces of milk a day that most well-fed mothers produce.

Fat-soluble pollutants are another reason to steer clear of diets. Because of pervasive pollution of the environment, nearly all of us have measurable levels of such poisons as DDT, chlordane, dieldrin, and even PCBs in our blood. The toxins accumulate in fatty tissue, including breast tissue. But so long as you don't fast or lose weight rapidly, they will stay in your own fatty tissue, they won't accumulate in your breast milk. Sudden weight loss—a melting away of fat—will release these poisons into your blood, and into your milk.

WHAT SUPPLEMENTS SHOULD YOU TAKE WHILE BREAST-FEEDING?

As nutritional insurance, you should continue with the supplements recommended for pregnant women (see p. 44). There are some important exceptions though.

- *Watch your intake of vitamin B-6.* With so many apparently healthy people being deficient in vitamin B-6,[4] probably because of our exposure to herbicides and other environmental B-6 antagonists (pp. 13, 42), it is not surprising perhaps that breast-feeding mothers must supplement their diets with 20 milligrams a day of vitamin B-6 just to make sure their infants receive the RDA of this vitamin.[5] On the other hand, excess vitamin B-6 (at levels of 200 milligrams a day or more) can inhibit lactation. If you have difficulty producing enough milk, cut B-6 back to 10 milligrams a day.
- *Eliminate the manganese supplement.* During your baby's first four to six weeks, her brain is exceptionally susceptible to the toxic effects of this mineral. Excess manganese is suspected of contributing to the later development of hyperactivity in youngsters. (See also the data on high manganese formulas, pp. 65–66.)

The amounts of most other vitamins and minerals in breast milk will not increase above normal levels even if you take large amounts as supplements. These include vitamins C, K, and B-3, folic acid and biotin, and the minerals sodium, calcium, zinc, fluorine, copper, and iron. Taking these in supplements will build up your own body's stores, but will not affect your baby.

If you take in enough iron during pregnancy, your baby will be born with enough in his bone marrow and liver to be in good health. But you should be aware that by the time your breast-fed child is nine or ten months old, these stores of iron may be used up. Luckily, by that time most babies are ready for foods that contain iron.

WHAT *NOT* TO TAKE WHILE BREAST-FEEDING

The last thing you will want to do is to transmit any toxins to your baby through your breast milk. Consult your physician before taking any drugs while breast-feeding. In particular, avoid every item on the following short list of drugs, drinks, additives, and other substances.

DRUGS

Opiates (including cough syrups with codeine and the pain-killer Demerol). If you *must* take such medications, be sure *not* to nurse your infant for at least *four hours* afterward.

Tranquilizers, whether *barbiturates* or *benzodiazepines* such as Valium or Librium.

Aspirin can interfere with your baby's normal blood-clotting activity—avoid it. If for some reason you *must* take it, don't breast-feed for four hours afterward.

Tylenol can damage your infant's liver.

Cough syrups containing iodine can affect your baby's thyroid function. You don't have to worry about the iodine in shellfish, though.

Caffeine is actually a drug, because the body becomes addicted to it. It can cause irritability and sleeplessness in your infant as well as yourself.

Nicotine is also a drug—don't smoke. The nicotine in cigarette tobacco can affect your baby's heartrate and produce vomiting and diarrhea.

Alcohol, even in small quantities, can damage your baby's brain cells. Drink fruit juice or seltzer instead.

Illegal drugs such as *marijuana* and *cocaine* can interfere with the functioning of your infant's developing brain.

FOOD / DRINK

Chocolate contains theobromine, easily transmitted in breast milk. It can make your infant irritable.

ADDITIVES

Aspartame, called NutraSweet, can be toxic to newborns, making them hyperexcitable. Some experiments with animals suggest that it may cause brain damage as well.

ENVIRONMENTAL POLLUTANTS

Pesticides are fat soluble and therefore easily transmitted in breast milk. (They enter your milk before being stored in your own body fat.) Large amounts of PCB herbicides (such as Agent Orange) have been identified in the milk of young mothers in many countries, including the United States. What can you do? First, avoid obvious large pesticide exposures. Cancel your contract with the exterminator and with the chemical lawn-care company (in addition to fertilizing your lawn, they treat it with weed- and bug killers). Safe ways to deal with pests, weeds, and other household problems are presented in the book *Nontoxic and Natural,* by Debra Lynn Dadd (1984). Even if you're not yet breast-feeding or are finished with it, the recommendations in that book offer health-promoting alternatives to contemporary causes of household pollution.

Second, do not diet while breast-feeding. The pesticides and herbicides that you have unknowingly consumed and inhaled for most of your life are stored in your body's fat tissue, where they are relatively harmless. Stringent diets that promote brisk weight loss release these stored toxins into your blood, increasing their concentration in your milk. When nursing your baby, you should eat heartily, not only to ensure good nutritional quality for your milk, but to keep pesticides out.

When Should You Not Breast-Feed?

There are two conditions under which breast-feeding can be harmful to your baby. If you are taking drugs to treat a disease, check with your doctor about their potential toxicity for your infant. If your baby has a disease, ask your pediatrician whether breast-feeding might adversely affect him. The commonest condition that can be made worse by breast milk is jaundice of the newborn. Jaundice is a yellow discoloration of skin and eyes caused by the accumulation of a natural chemical called bilirubin in the blood. Normally, the liver excretes bilirubin into the bile, but in many newborns the liver is unable to do this efficiently at the time of birth. In older infants and children, bilirubin itself is nontoxic, although jaundice may be a sign of serious disease. In newborns, jaundice is not usually a sign of disease, just of age, but bilirubin can be toxic to the brain if high enough blood levels are reached. Breast milk contains substances that can slow the excretion of bilirubin by the liver. If your newborn infant has serious jaundice, such that hospitalization or medical therapy is being contemplated, see if a temporary cessation of breast-feeding (one to two weeks should be enough) allows the condition to improve.[6]

HOW TO MANAGE THE WORKING MOTHER'S OPTIONS
Breast-Feeding Full Time or Part Time and How to Manage If You Can't Breast-Feed at All

HOW DO YOU BREAST-FEED FULL TIME AND STILL HOLD DOWN A JOB?

It's not easy, but it can be done. There are three possible options:

Do both at once. This is the hardest one. If you are lucky enough to have the kind of work situation that permits it, you can bring your baby to work with you and breast-feed there. But even if your co-workers are enormously supportive, it can be exhausting to try to give 100 percent to both your baby and your job.

Adjust your job to your baby's needs. This is a popular solution, but it's not always possible. It depends on the kind of work you do. By working part time, or sharing a job with someone else, though, you can breast-feed full time without sacrificing the energy you need for your job and your baby.

Adjust your baby's nursing to your full-time job. This is the most prevalent solution, but it means that you will have to express your milk into sterile containers and refrigerate or freeze it. Your care giver can then bottle-feed your breast milk to your baby while you are at work.

The catch is that most women can express only a few ounces of milk at a time, whereas a baby needs 4 ounces per feeding. This means you will have to express milk several times to accumulate enough for a baby's needs while you are at work.

A Schedule for Breast-Feeding When You Work Full Time

This has worked for many mothers.

Morning. Get up about an hour earlier than you normally do. This gives you 15 minutes for your own needs. Use the next 45 minutes in these segments:

10 minutes to breast-feed on one side;
10 minutes to burp and hold your baby;
10 minutes to breast-feed the other side; and
15 minutes to gently pat, burp, and cradle your baby to sleep (you hope).

Lunchtime. Breast-feeding during the day is only practical if you live near your work. You can go home to breast-feed at lunchtime, or, if you have the option, have your care giver bring the baby to you at work for breast-feeding in your private office or a comfortable corner of the women's lounge, assuming you have the former or the latter exists, and you can arrange the time. If you nurse in your private office, you may find co-workers who barge in on you nonplussed at first. One mother reports that she hangs a sign on her door to warn colleagues to wait a few minutes.

If you don't live close enough to work to make breast-feeding practical, your care giver will give your baby a warmed bottle of refrigerated or frozen breast milk.

After Work. Tell your sitter or day-care center worker what time you expect to get home so that he or she won't feed your baby for at least an hour before you arrive. That way, you can feed your baby as soon as you get home. If you expect to be delayed, ask the care giver to feed the baby some cooled-down (warm to the touch) boiled water.

You may find it helpful to breast-feed your baby two or three times after you arrive home, including, if you wish, once just before bed. This helps her to feel full and sleepy by the time you are ready for bed yourself.

When Can You Express Your Milk?

You can express an ounce of milk in about five minutes, and in an average feeding your baby will take in about four ounces. If you have enough milk, you can express some milk just before feeding your baby in the morning and evening. You can also express enough milk over a weekend for your baby to drink while you are at work during the week. If you can arrange the privacy, you can express milk during the workday, but only if you can refrigerate it until you get home. (In fact, when you breast-feed, your breasts will tend to fill with milk every two hours, so you will feel more comfortable if you can express milk or nurse during the day.)

You can express your milk either manually or with a breast pump. For instructions on how to do this, I highly recommend Sally Wendkos Olds's *The Complete Book of Breastfeeding.*

Breast milk is highly perishable; refrigerate or freeze it in sterile containers. (I prefer not to use plastic bags because substances in the plastic that keep it soft can dissolve in the fat of the milk and will be consumed by your infant. These plastic softeners have been shown to cause cancer in experimental animals.) Sterilize glass jars by boiling them in water for twenty minutes. Let them cool from hot to warm, then fill with breast milk and refrigerate or freeze. Refrigerated breast milk will keep for twenty-four hours; frozen, it will keep for up to thirty days.

You can add fresh breast milk to a partially full container of frozen milk and return the container to the freezer, but only if you add less than the amount already frozen. If you add more, the fresh warm milk will thaw the frozen. In so doing, it may change its quality and allow bacteria to grow.

USING A FORMULA

If it's not possible to breast-feed full time with any of the arrangements above, it's still better to breast-feed part time than not at all. And that means your care giver will feed your child a formula while you're at work. *If at all possible, though, do try to breast-feed full time for her first six weeks of life.* There are no perfect formulas for very young infants, either in terms of nutrition or of immune protection. Infants under six weeks are especially susceptible to infections; they need the protection breast milk provides.

Infant formulas are all contaminated with aluminum, a toxic metal, and contain 30 to 100 times as much aluminum as breast milk.[7] In infants with kidney disease, formula feeding can cause brain damage from aluminum toxicity. The effect of aluminum on normal newborns is not known.

If you are unable to breast-feed at all, you will have to supplement your baby's formula to compensate for its lack of EFAs and antioxidants. After I've discussed formulas, I will provide detailed information on how to supplement them.

What About Cow's or Goat's Milk? I don't believe children should have cow's milk until they're a year old. Many infants are allergic to it because their digestive tracts haven't developed enough to be able to handle it. Studies show that the overabundant casein in cow's milk can curdle. The result? Your baby feels discomfort and spits up the milk.

Goat's milk is a fair *occasional* substitute for breast milk, but it's too low in folic acid and vitamin B-12 to be adequate as your child's sole food. While it's not so overrich in protein as cow's milk, it still has much more than human breast milk, and must be diluted two to one with water. Since, unlike breast milk, it isn't sterile, it has to be boiled.

Milk-Based Formulas. Although they have their drawbacks, milk-based formulas are the best and most convenient substitutes for breast milk. Processing renders their protein less allergenic, but look for a formula that lists added whey. Whey and casein are different components of milk. Casein is harder to digest and more allergenic than whey, and, as I pointed out above, cow's milk contains more casein than human milk. Added whey means the ratio of whey and casein in the formula has been adjusted to approximate that of breast milk.

A high manganese content is a serious problem with some

formulas, because newborns may be particularly susceptible to the toxic effects of excess manganese. Many learning-disabled children have higher than normal amounts of manganese in their hair, and although we don't know whether the cause is excessive absorption of manganese or too much manganese in food, the problem may start in the first few months of life.[8]

For the first three months, a formula should be low in iron, too, to avoid the risk of gastroenteritis. (See p. 54 for a discussion of the problems infants have with iron.) In fact, for the first four months, look for a formula that's low in both manganese and iron. After that, switch to one that is iron-fortified.

The following list compares three widely available milk-based formulas. Note that all are low in magnesium, but two are high in manganese. Also note that when you sterilize a formula, you inevitably destroy some of the added vitamins, among them C and B-6.

BRAND	GOOD FEATURE	BAD FEATURE
Enfamil	added whey added taurine or high iron	100 mcg/liter of manganese, three times that of human milk low magnesium
Similac	low manganese (same amount as breast milk) comes with low or high iron	no whey low magnesium
Sma	added whey	high manganese low magnesium

Recommendation. Because Similac is low in manganese, it is probably the best choice. However, it contains no added whey to offset the heavy casein content. If your child cannot digest it, try Enfamil as second choice.

Soy Formulas. I don't recommend any of these because they are low in *carnitine,* a substance essential for proper fat metabolism. They are useful for children who are allergic to cow's milk formulas, while providing approximately the same nutrition. But they contain up to nine times more manganese than breast milk.

Some Tips on Formula Feeding

- *Check the lead content of your water supply.* Ask your water department for the statistics, or have your water checked by a private laboratory. (Try running the cold water for three or more minutes in the morning to flush out any lead leached in overnight from solder on pipe joints.) If it has a lead content greater than 0.03 parts per million, use a ready-to-feed formula that doesn't require added water, or use bottled spring water in preparing formula.
- *If you use tap water, boil it uncovered for five minutes before adding it to the formula.* This will kill germs and help evaporate the chlorine added to all tap water.
- *Never, ever, give a bottle to a sleeping child.* While she may feed in her sleep by reflex, problems are likely. At worst, she can choke. Also, feeding during sleep encourages bacteria in the mouth to form lactic acid, which rots developing teeth.

Compensating for a Formula's Nutritional Deficits

All formulas are inadequate in GLA and omega-3 EFA, and Similac contains no added taurine. If you breast-feed part time, and you are well-nourished, your milk will compensate for these inadequacies. If you can't breast-feed at all, you should supplement the formula. Fortunately, this isn't hard to do.

GLA. One best source is Efamol (brand) evening primrose oil. It comes in 500-milligram capsules. Another source is black currant oil, which usually comes in 250-milligram capsules. Once a day, rub the oil from one capsule of either oil into your baby's skin. It will be absorbed into her body. (See p. 19 for a complete discussion of evening primrose oil and other sources of EFAs.) *Under no circumstances should you try to get a child under four years old to swallow a capsule.*

Omega-3 EFA. The best source is the organically grown flaxseed oil from Omega Nutrition, found in health-food stores or by writing to Omega Nutrition, 165–810 West Broadway, Vancouver, British Columbia V5ZYC9, or Allergy Resources, Box 2131, Port Washington, N.Y. 11050. Your baby can take a total of 1

teaspoon a day in her formula, divided among three feedings. Add
⅓ teaspoon to a bottle before sterilization. If your baby has no
problem with it, try adding the whole teaspoonful at once. If
flaxseed oil is not available, use 4 drops of cod-liver oil three times
a day or ⅓ tablespoon of walnut oil three times a day. Oils contain
no protein, so they are not major allergens. (See p. 17 for a complete discussion of flaxseed oil and other sources of EFAs.)

You can also rub flaxseed or walnut oil into her skin. In India,
infants are regularly anointed with oil as part of a ritual of love
and tenderness. A teaspoon of flaxseed or walnut oil will anoint
your infant's entire body. Don't use more than that. The oil will
be absorbed on its own; you don't need to rub it all in.

Two important warnings about flaxseed oil:

- *It should have almost no taste. If it tastes even slightly bitter
  it is rancid; throw it out.*
- *Never use boiled linseed oil that is made from flaxseeds from
  the hardware or paint store. It is poison.*

Taurine. Enfamil has enough taurine. You can bring the
taurine content of Similac up to that of breast milk by sprinkling
about one-fourth of a 500-milligram capsule of taurine into each
quart of formula before sterilization. Vital-life, Nutricology, and
Tyson are reputable brands of the L-taurine I recommend. They
are available at health-food stores.

HOW TO HANDLE FEEDING PROBLEMS

- *I can't tell whether my child is cranky, hungry, or sick. Does
  every cry mean I should feed my baby?*

A whimper doesn't mean distress or hunger—you don't have
to nurse your baby continually. A sudden strong cry, or wail,
usually means your infant is uncomfortable, but a small tired cry
may just mean some temporary irritation. If you think your child
is cranky but not hungry, try changing her diaper, or even just
talking or singing to her in a quiet, soothing voice.

Life is made harder for working mothers by the fact that
most children get fussy and need attention around 6:00 P.M. So if
you are rushing home from work every night to be with your
child, you will be asked to drop your own needs the minute you

arrive—even though that's just when you need some quiet moments yourself.

Drs. Urs Hunziker and Ronald Barr of Montreal Children's Hospital found that infant-carrying practices play a large role in determining the irritability of young infants and may account for the greater frequency of crying among babies in industrial countries than is found in traditional, preindustrial cultures. In industrial societies, a crying infant can become an incessant problem for some parents, eroding coping skills and possibly contributing to child abuse. Crying tends to peak about the sixth week. In a study that compared the effect of extra carrying with other forms of attention, Drs. Hunziker and Barr found that two hours a day of extra carrying during the first three months of life produced a 43 percent decrease in crying and fussing, increased "awake contentment" as reported by the mothers, and eliminated the six-week crying peak. A Snuggly or similar chest or back carrier is a handy way to accomplish this, and can be used by your spouse or care giver as well. Not only will you increase "carrying time," you will increase physical contact with your baby and become more attuned to his moods and movements. If carrying the baby hurts your back, look for Sarah's Ride, a hip carrier.

Your child's color and temperature will tell you whether she is really sick. As long as she's pink, she's probably fine. If she turns blue, gray, or blotchy, she's probably ill. Suddenly cold hands and feet may indicate a problem, too.

Here are some other signals to look for.

Signs of mild dehydration. Are her eyes and mouth dry? Does her skin seem dry and less elastic than when she is well?

A lack of responsiveness. Does she fail to respond to your smiles, gestures, and cuddling? Does she seem bored with her toys?

A different kind of cry. Her crying may sound angrier, more intense, more distraught.

Excessive sleepiness. Is she sleeping more than usual? Do you have a hard time waking her up?

Glassy eyes. Just as you do when you have a cold or the flu, your infant may become glassy-eyed when she is sick.

- *What do I do if she is sick and doesn't want to eat?* When your
infant is sick, she will need less food than usual; never force
food on her. But if she seems dehydrated (see above), give her
water to drink. If she has a cold and is dripping mucus, you can
use a nasal saltwater wash to dissolve it. Add ⅛ teaspoon of
regular table salt or coarse salt to half a glass (about 4 ounces)
of boiled, cooled-down water. Use the tip of a baby enema syringe to squirt this solution *into the edge* (not up) of the nostril.
If you have no baby enema syringe, dip a clean, soft cotton
handkerchief into the salt water, wring it out, and gently wipe
away the mucus.
- *What if I have a cold or sore throat? Should I stop breast-
feeding and keep away from my baby?* No! Keep right on
breast-feeding—just take some precautions. Wash your hands
carefully before you go near the baby, and, if you like, you can
wear a respiratory mask or a handkerchief when you hold her.

  For a cold, take a lot of fluids—water, orange juice, hot
chicken soup, herbal teas. And this is the time for megadoses of
vitamin C: 1,000 to 3,000 milligrams every hour. If you get a touch
of diarrhea, you will know you have reached your limit of tolerance and you can lower your dosage. These megadoses won't get
into your breast milk, so you don't have to worry about affecting
your baby.

  For a sore throat, I always find it helpful to keep my throat
warm and gargle with salt water. Zinc lozenges (no more than five
a day) can relieve pain. Hot lemonade made with fresh lemon juice
and a touch of honey is an old and effective remedy. As with a cold,
drink lots of liquids and take megadoses of vitamin C.
- *If my baby has colic, could my diet be responsible?* I've long
thought that colic in breast-fed babies might have something to
do with the mother's consumption of cow's milk. Swedish doctors studied eighteen mothers of colicky babies who eliminated
milk from their diets. In thirteen of the babies, the colic disappeared.

  Also watch for hard-to-digest foods or drinks, as these are apt
to be passed along to the baby in breast milk. Avoid such gas-
producing foods as beans, lentils, brussels sprouts, broccoli, cabbage, mushrooms, sodas, and, of course, alcohol. Also watch
spices! Recently, a young mother reported to me that she had
gleefully gone out for her first restaurant meal after her baby's

birth. "We went to a wonderful Mexican restaurant," she told me. "I certainly learned a lesson about spices! Paavo was sick and irritable for the next twenty-four hours!"

- *My baby seems too hungry for the amount of milk my breasts can supply—or she doesn't seem to grow well on breast milk alone.* Remember, infants are hungry frequently—in fact, it's natural for everyone, adults as well as infants, to want to feed every ninety minutes. Three meals a day is simply a convention that allows society to get its work done. So if your baby is hungry often, that doesn't necessarily mean your milk is inadequate. If she isn't growing as fast as she should, your pediatrician will advise you to supplement your own milk with a formula. But as long as breast-feeding remains her major source of nourishment, she will still benefit from all the special nutrients in your milk.

  Unfortunately, there is no magic formula for increasing the amount of milk you are able to supply. You will produce more if you are relaxed and calm, if you eat about 1,900 calories a day, breast-feed frequently, and watch your intake of vitamin B-6, for it could interfere with lactation. Don't take more than 30 milligrams of vitamin B-6 a day. If you are breast-feeding part time, you will probably keep up a better flow of milk if you breast-feed at night rather than giving your baby a bottle.

- *How will I know when it's time to wean her?* There is no "right age" for weaning a baby. Ideally, your baby will wean herself, sometime after eleven months. As she learns to love solid foods, she will feed less frequently at your breast. You can encourage her to wean herself by feeding her solid foods more frequently, which brings us to the question of how to introduce your baby to solid foods.

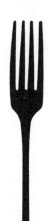

Six Months to a Year: Building Up Young Bodies When Starting Solid Food

4

At some point between his fourth and seventh month, a baby is ready to start eating solid food. Don't rush this moment; for both your sakes, it's better for him to start solid food later rather than earlier. The best thing to do is to let him tell you when he's ready: He will be able to sit up well and he will seem hungrier than usual between his feedings. A sure sign is that he will begin moving his tongue back and forth in his mouth, rather than up and down in the sucking pattern. This means he is ready to move food from his lips to his throat.

There are some very good reasons not to rush your baby into solid food:

- When he starts eating solid foods, the wonderful, protective *Lactobacillus bifidus* will disappear from his intestinal tract. At seven months, he will be better able to handle this loss than at four months.

- Assuming you've been breast-feeding, the extra couple of months of breast milk will help sustain and enhance his developing immune system, minimizing any chance of food allergies.[1] Allergenic reactions will increase the susceptibility of his intestinal and respiratory tracts to infection, just at the point when he is susceptible anyway because he is losing his *bifidus* protection.

- It's much more convenient for you, because at seven months he can handle mashed food; you won't have to purée or strain everything.

On the other hand, I don't see any reason to prolong exclusive breast-feeding much past seven months. A century ago, babies were given no solids until they were a year old, which wasn't a bad idea at the time. Hygiene was relatively poor and the incidence of intestinal-tract infections was high. But my experience is that babies are physiologically ready for solid foods at seven months.

At that age, the limitations of breast milk start to become significant, too. It is low in iron and vitamin D, and may not provide enough calories or protein for an older baby's growth. So, although I advocate nothing but breast milk for his first six months, at seven months it is definitely time for solid food.

Here are some common questions mothers often ask me about this transition:

- *Can you prevent food allergies if you breast-feed exclusively for a full year?* Unfortunately, breast milk only delays the onset of food allergies; it can't prevent them altogether. Good nutrition, with special attention to EFAs, will do a good deal more to prevent allergies than delaying solid foods.
- *How can you tell if you've started solid foods too soon?* If he spits them out, or drools when he's fed, he's probably not ready; wait a few more weeks. Don't try to force him to eat; stop feeding as soon as he stops eating.
- *What if he resists spoon feeding?* Many babies go through this stage, either because they want to keep sucking or because they want to feed themselves. Don't force-feed him; it will just build frustration and increase resistance. I don't advise adding sugar to his food either; that will just accustom him to overly sweet foods and contribute to tooth decay. If he wants to suck, let him breast-feed longer. When he gets hungry enough so that breast milk no longer suffices, he will start to accept solids.

If he doesn't want to let you put the spoon into his mouth, and grasps at the spoon or the food—or both—you'll know he wants to feed himself. If he's able to grasp with his fingers, he may be ready to feed himself at least some of the time. But if he grasps with his palm, he's not ready.

What to do? Give him thick, sticky foods that he can grasp with his palm and put into his mouth: big lumps of thick, cold baby cereal or moistened, fork-mashed potatoes; mashed vegetables stuck together with oatmeal, or pieces of peeled fruit. This kind of food gives him a more varied diet than milk alone, and helps him develop the pincer grasp that will enable him to hold a spoon.

At first he will play with his food more than he'll eat it. But if he eats with his parents or siblings, their example and his own hunger should have him eating more and playing less before your patience runs out.

HOW TO INTRODUCE YOUR BABY TO SOLID FOODS

WHAT TO START WITH

Until now, your baby has had nothing but liquids with a fairly limited range of tastes. Now he is ready for cereal, fruits, and vegetables (high-protein foods come later). You won't want to overwhelm him with new tastes and textures. A good rule of thumb is to introduce new foods to him one at a time.

Giving him a larger amount of a single food at a feeding, rather than small amounts of several foods, allows him to get used to a new food so that he'll be less likely to reject it. He'll also be less likely to have an allergic reaction. Strange as it seems, a small amount of a new food is more likely to induce his immune system to form allergic antibodies than is a larger amount.

You will want to start him on soft, bland, smooth foods, such as cereal. Then, over a period of four to six months, he can learn to accept different tastes and textures while he develops chewing skills and learns to feed himself. When he's mastered cereal, you can add foods with a coarser texture and stronger taste, such as squash. Cooking and puréeing will make even such vegetables as beans suitable until he is ready for chunky, chewy foods such as broccoli. Last of all come finger foods such as cooked carrot sticks. By this time, your baby will be ready to start eating his meals at the table with the rest of the family. (But it's not necessary to name his meals or worry about what he eats at what time of day. At this point, it's all just food to him.)

His First Solid Food: Iron-Fortified Cereal

You will want to start your baby off on iron-fortified rice, oat, or barley cereal. No wheat until he's a year old, because it's more likely to produce an allergic reaction.

The iron is important because by this time your child's iron stores are used up, and he needs iron so that his brain will develop properly. Studies have shown that children who are only mildly iron-deficient—so mildly that they aren't anemic—score lower on tests of mental function than control children. Correcting the iron deficiency improves mental performance.[2]

Iron will also prevent anemia and enable his body to resist infection. Contrary to a popular belief, an iron deficiency at this age will not protect a baby against infection. In fact, it can only do him harm. As we saw in the last chapter, it is only newborn infants who have problems with iron. (Older children and adults with *serious* protein deficiencies are unable to use iron, either, but that is another story.)

Furthermore, iron deficiency increases the absorption of lead from food.[3] Increases in the blood lead level, even within the so-called safe range, adversely affects the intellectual function and school achievement of children.[4] Lead enters food through processing (lead solder in cans) and from house dust.[5]

Preparing Your Baby's Cereal. Use breast milk or formula as the liquid. You will want to start with a consistency only slightly thicker than milk. As your child becomes able to handle it, you can gradually thicken it to the more usual consistency. A good method is to start with a thin cereal broth and gradually add more cereal to get the texture you want. Feed a very small amount—about ⅛ teaspoon—at a time, slowly increasing the amount as he is able to handle it.

Every three days or so, he should be ready for a new cereal. A good order is a rice cereal, then oatmeal, then a barley cereal. If you use a dry cereal, you will of course soak it thoroughly until it is soft, then dilute it to the right consistency.

Food #2: Vegetables

Once your baby is happily eating cereals, he's ready to meet vegetables. Start with puréed green beans and peas, pumpkin, squash, and potatoes, both sweet and white.

Don't give your baby spinach, beets, turnips, carrots, or collard greens until he is nine months old. While they are excellent sources of important nutrients, especially vitamin A, these vegetables may be too rich in nitrates for him before that. Nitrates can change his red blood cells so that they are less able to carry oxygen.

Food #3: Fruits

About a month after starting vegetables, he should be ready to tackle fruits. I recommend applesauce, peaches, apricots, pears, nectarines, and plums. Avoid bananas—their porous skin admits the toxic fungicides that, by law, must be sprayed on all imported fruits. (In general, avoid any imported fruits, but bananas are the most dangerous. They are not so problematic for older children, but infants' immature livers are ill-prepared to detoxify and eliminate pesticides. Older, heavier children, whose livers function better, will not be harmed by an occasional piece of imported fruit.) To be on the safe side, *use only washed or peeled local fruits in season.* Out-of-season fruit may well be imported. Buy ripened fruits—they're tastiest and most nutritious, and are the easiest to mash or purée.

Start with cooked fruit; it's easiest to bake it. Preheat the oven to 350°F. Wash the fruit. To preserve its nutrients, bake it in its skin in a covered dish with just a little water. When it's tender, it's done. You can also steam it in a tightly covered pot. Either way, peel before puréeing or mashing. You probably won't have to add water for a smooth purée, since both cooking methods preserve natural liquids as well as nutrients. If you must add water, use the absolute minimum.

When your child can handle cooked fruit, try uncooked mashed fruit. The chewier texture will help him learn to chew. If he has a good grasp and chew, you can give him small pieces to hold, chew, and suck on. *Caution:* he must be able to chew well, mashing the fruit on his own, or he might choke on hard fruit, such as apple or pear.

Food #4: More Vegetables

Once he's mastered fruits, your baby is ready for chewier vegetables: zucchini, broccoli, cauliflower, asparagus tips, kale, and tomatoes. (Although they are soft and easily puréed, he wasn't ready for tomatoes earlier because of their acidity and strong taste.)

He's also old enough now to eat spinach, beets, turnips, carrots, and collard greens. Serve each one every four to five days until he becomes familiar with them. Don't make the servings too large. If he shows gassiness or bloating, especially after eating turnips or collard greens, wait about a month before trying them again.

TIPS ON FOOD PREPARATION

- *It's best to prepare your baby's food yourself.* These days, with a blender or food processor, or both, in almost every home, it's easy to purée fresh vegetables. It's also simple to strain them. Either way is fine.
- *Leave out the sugar, salt, or fat.* These anti-nutrients do nothing for your baby, and, as we saw in Chapter 1, they slow down EFA metabolism. And *that* distorts the production line of prostaglandins, the chemicals that keep the immune system running properly. Anti-nutrients also increase the body's need for certain nutrients: sugar demands more vitamin B for its metabolism, while salt increases the amount of magnesium lost in the urine.

  Babies love sweet foods, but they can get all the sweetness they want from fruits. If you add sugar, you're just adding empty calories while discouraging your child from acquiring more subtle tastes.

  Never give honey to a child who is less than a year old. It could be contaminated with spores from botulism-causing bacteria. The Centers for Disease Control, the national disease clearinghouse in Atlanta, has reported infant deaths from botulism poisoning because of contaminated honey.

  The desire for added salt is an acquired taste. Your baby won't think unsalted foods are bland; to him, they'll be interesting new tastes.

Commercial Baby Foods

There are some good-quality commercial products on the market, but be sure to check the labels to see that they don't contain additives of any sort—don't buy any that list sugar, salt, BHT or BHA (preservatives that may be allergenic or toxic), or EDTA, a color-preserving agent that binds to minerals such as calcium and magnesium, preventing their absorption. EDTA, sugar, and salt are all anti-nutrients.

Years ago, baby-food manufacturers routinely added sugar and salt to please a mother's taste buds. Today, though, Beechnut and some other major producers offer natural baby foods, free of sugar, salt, and preservatives. These products are sterile and nutritionally about as good as the food you prepare yourself. Note, though, that the chances are that any baby food labeled "dessert" has been sweetened.

Buy food in jars, not cans—canned baby foods may be contaminated by the lead used to solder the seams. Choose "single" foods rather than "dinners" combining different foods. In addition to containing more than one food, the dinners are more likely to contain added fat and salt.

TEN MONTHS: PROTEIN TIME

Until now, your infant's kidneys and digestive tract were not ready to handle high-protein foods. But these foods are rich in vitamins and minerals, too, and your baby is finally ready to take advantage of them.

At this point, he will be getting most of his nutrition from solid foods. He is ready for meat, poultry, beans, egg yolks (save the whites for another couple of months; they can be allergenic at this stage), and tofu, or bean curd. This last, an easy-to-use form of the highly nutritious soybean, is found in many stores today.

Beans work best when combined with grains to produce a more complete protein. Many cultures around the world have evolved staple dishes of this combination: rice and beans in Latin America, corn and lima beans, known to us as succotash, among Native Americans, sesame seeds and chick-peas in the Middle

East. For a baby, make hummus—sesame butter (tahini) and ground chick-peas.

Seeds and nuts are also rich in proteins, vitamins, and minerals—and EFAs as well. Nut butters are easy to make and your infant will enjoy them from now on through his childhood (see p. 261 for the recipe). If you like, you can purée meat and poultry from your table for him. Skip fish, though, until he is a year old. Like egg whites, they are likely to be allergenic.

Finger-lickin' good. One of the many nice things about being ten months old is enjoying real finger foods. Give him pieces of fresh peeled, pitted fruit, tofu chunks, or small pieces of moist cooked chicken. (These are bigger, chewier foods than the small, soft pieces of fruit you may have given him earlier.)

EFAs. To be sure your baby is getting enough of the all-important omega-3 EFAs, it's a good idea to add about a teaspoon of food-grade flaxseed oil or 1 tablespoon of walnut oil to his meals each day. You can mix it into meat and vegetable dishes.

The best quality of unrefined flaxseed oil is made by Omega Nutrition. Taste it before using. It should have virtually no taste, although some people detect a very slight fishy aftertaste. If it tastes bitter, it is rancid; throw it out.

ONE YEAR OLD: THE OMNIVOROUS EATER

At this age, your baby can eat almost anything. He has a few teeth, so he can chew more, and his digestive system can handle whole milk, whole eggs, yogurt, fish, and wheat. He will want to feed himself, and you should encourage him to do so as much as possible. You will still have to cut up his food, but he can pick up the pieces with his hands and put them in his mouth. He may miss occasionally, but he'll learn. By this time, he should be eating at the table with the rest of the family.

In the joy of eating, there is one danger: foods that can slip down his windpipe. He's not really ready yet for whole nuts, raw carrots (the small chunks he bites off can create trouble), or popcorn. These won't be safe for him to eat until he is about eighteen months old.

Serving Suggestions. Among cereals, Wheatena is the best addition to his diet now; it's made of nutritious, unrefined whole grains. Cream of Wheat is not a whole-grain product, so it's less nutritious. He's still not ready for dry cereals, though.

You can crumble whole wheat toast into very small pieces and soak it in milk. You can also purée cooked whole wheat pasta in a small amount of milk.

Mash fish after removing both skin and bones.

Give your baby at this stage of life plain, whole-milk yogurt rather than cow's milk. Yogurt is more digestible, and adds beneficial lactobacillus organisms to his intestinal tract. You can mix fresh fruit with it, but stay away from the commercial high-sugar, yogurt-with-fruit combinations. Many of them contain pre-servatives, as well. Your child will enjoy plain yogurt all his life if he acquires a taste for it now.

DOES HE NEED SUPPLEMENTS?

The chances are that your pediatrician will already have your baby on a multivitamin with fluoride. I don't believe that a healthy infant who is eating well needs any supplement except linseed oil. And I have serious reservations about the use of fluorides (see the section on tooth care that follows this one). Nevertheless, such supplements are probably harmless.

If your child is prone to infections, he will need more than the average multivitamin. Give him the following every day:

Vitamin C	200 mg
Folic acid	400 mcg (.04 mg)
Iron	10 mg
Zinc	5 mg

Vitamin D is actually not a vitamin at all—it's a hormone formed in the body by the action of sunlight. There is very little vitamin D in breast milk or cow's milk, although the latter is usually vitamin-D fortified. But the best source of D is still sun-light.

It doesn't take much; fifteen minutes a day at midday, sum-mer or winter, even fully clothed, is enough. The sun on his hands and face will do the job. In the early morning or late afternoon, double the time. In the south, he needs less time; in the north, a bit more.

Children whose skin is dark, or those who live in the far north, may have a problem getting enough sun during the winter. They can take 100 milligrams of infant vitamin D every day. Older children shouldn't need a supplement because so many commercial foods (including meat) have been directly or indirectly fortified with vitamin D. (Animal feed is laced with it.)

HOW TO START HIS TEETH OFF RIGHT

Tooth decay is endemic in children today, but you can do a lot to prevent it. Even before you can see your baby's teeth, they are right under the skin of his gums, and sugar, the worst culprit in tooth decay, can already begin to affect them. And even though you are keeping refined sugar, honey, and molasses out of his diet altogether, you still have to deal with the natural sugars in fruits and root vegetables. A few rules of thumb will help:

- *Never give your baby fruit juice in a bottle.* Wait until he can drink from a cup. When he sucks from a bottle, he bathes his mouth in sugar-laden fluids; when he drinks from a cup, the fluids leave his mouth more quickly.
- *Don't give him anything sweet before bedtime.* This includes fresh or dried fruit (preferably without added preservatives) or juice. During the day, his saliva continually washes his teeth and gums, carrying away sugars. But during sleep the saliva flow is much reduced, so sugars stay longer in the mouth.
- *Use a piece of clean gauze to wipe his teeth after every meal until he's old enough to begin brushing his teeth.*

What About Fluorides? Fluoride, whether occurring naturally in water or added as a supplement, can strengthen teeth against decay. But *too much* can inhibit the action of certain enzymes in your baby's blood as well as causing brown stains on his teeth. Tooth decay is caused by an excess of sugar, not a deficiency of fluoride; there is no evidence that fluoride supplements help prevent cavities if taken beyond the first year of life.

THE "INVISIBLE" NUTRIENT

When you breast-fed your baby, the two of you were close, both physically and emotionally, and the bond between you steadily deepened. As he was weaned, you still spent a lot of time with him, feeding him and touching him, and he was still very dependent on you.

Now that he is beginning to be more independent, there will be progressively fewer occasions when you must touch him to care for him. As he grows older, he will do more and more things for himself, but you will want to keep the warm love you have built strong and alive while he begins to build ties with the rest of the family. Meals are good occasions for building and reinforcing these family bonds; keep them easy, relaxed, and happy.

HOW TO COPE WITH HEALTH PROBLEMS DURING YOUR BABY'S FIRST YEAR

You can expect your baby to have minor problems during his first year of life—a cold or two, transient diarrhea, equally transient irritability. But if he develops health problems that persist for longer than three weeks, they may signify an underlying disturbance. The most common chronic problems at this age are colic, diarrhea, constipation, poor sleep, irritability, spitting up, congestion, cough, diaper rash, recurrent throat and ear infections, and eczema.

In my experience, these problems usually occur against a background of food allergies and certain nutritional deficiencies. The most common deficiencies involve magnesium and EFAs. In addition, a child with recurrent infections may have a zinc, iron, or vitamin A deficiency. If you follow my diet plan, your baby shouldn't have any dietary deficiencies, but some infants have trouble absorbing certain nutrients, or converting them to an active form.

In addition, a yeast, *Candida albicans*, can cause both severe diaper rash and thrush, a painful mouth infection. Infants are prone to *Candida* infections because their immune systems are immature. Antibiotics are often given to infants, sometimes inappropriately. These drugs kill normal bacteria in the intestine that prevent *Candida* from flourishing there. Once they are killed off, an overgrowth of yeast can lead to serious problems. *Candida* is a potent allergen, and *Candida*-induced allergies complicate the picture for many infants with chronic problems who have been given antibiotics.

Evaluating and treating any of these problems will involve one or more of the following:

More EFAs
More magnesium, sometimes with vitamins B-1 and B-6
For chronic infection, more iron, zinc, and vitamin A
A food-allergy evaluation
Oral Nystatin (an antifungal drug) and lactobacilli (the beneficial bacteria killed off by antibiotics, if a child has a yeast infection or a history of taking antibiotics)

In the pages that follow, I will take you step by step through the evaluation and treatment of these common chronic problems.

THE SYMPTOMS

Colic. He screams intensely, and he is not soothed by burping. He passes a great deal of gas and has abnormally hard or loose stools. He flexes his legs against his abdomen in an attempt to relieve the pain.

Diarrhea. Loose or watery movements lasting more than a few days.

Constipation. Rock-hard, pebbly stool, or bowel movements less often than every day.

Spitting Up. He spits up even familiar foods.

Excess Mucus, Coughing, or Congestion. If any of these problems lasts more than three weeks, it is usually food-related.

Severe Diaper Rash. Persistent angry redness of the skin.

Recurrent Throat and Ear Infection. See below, under Recurrent Infections, page 91.

Eczema. Red, scaling patches of skin anywhere on the body.

Behavioral Disturbances. Many temperamental children have been brought to me, usually after the age of one, by which time their problems have affected the whole family. Often these children are more alert, more inquisitive, and brighter than other youngsters their age. They may even have reached certain developmental milestones earlier. But their poor adaptability and their negative moods can make them very hard to live with.

Dr. Stanley Turecki of Mount Sinai Hospital in New York City has written an excellent book, *The Difficult Child* (1985), that lists some key traits that can be detected in infancy.

In general, everything—people, touch, noises, or music—seems to overstimulate him. He won't cuddle; when you try to hold him, he kicks and squirms a lot. Or he reacts to even gentle touching by withdrawing. It's hard to dress or bathe him.

He reacts to any unfamiliar noise as if it were a firecracker going off under his nose. He tends to be very loud himself, whether he is happy or sad.

He is restless, fussy, cranky, or irritable much of the time and he sleeps irregularly and restlessly. He hates any change in routine. He eats on an irregular schedule, and reacts to new foods by spitting them out.

If any of these traits persist for over a month, you can consider them chronic.

THE MAGNESIUM CONNECTION IN COLIC AND BEHAVIORAL PROBLEMS

The first step for young infants should be to increase carrying time (see above p. 69). If colic or temperamental behavior become chronic, your baby might need magnesium supplementation, especially if he's over six months old. As I said above, if you are following my diet, your infant is unlikely to have a magnesium deficiency, but he might have trouble absorbing the mineral. This *creates* a deficiency that, in turn, affects calcium-regulating hormones. The result is a calcium deficiency. And that can cause intestinal spasms and irritability.

Babies with behavioral problems generally require more magnesium than do other infants—perhaps because the hormones secreted during their chronic high levels of stress trigger greater than normal excretion of magnesium in their urine.

In either case, 100 to 200 milligrams of magnesium a day should help. You will soon know if the dose is too high because excess magnesium causes diarrhea. If that happens, simply cut back on the amount of magnesium, 50 milligrams at a time, until his stools are normal again.

Two inexpensive, easily available sources of magnesium are *magnesium citrate* and *milk of magnesia:* 100 milligrams of magnesium = ½ teaspoon magnesium citrate, or ½ teaspoon milk of magnesia.

Add a tiny amount to his food at each feeding, making sure the total reaches ½ to 1 teaspoon a day but does not exceed that amount. Magnesium generally has a calming effect and enhances sleep, a bonus in both colic and behavioral problems.

If magnesium supplements help with colic, sleep, or reduce irritability, I would continue them. The purest source for long-term use is magnesium citrate capsules. Magnesium citrate liquid and milk of magnesia often have artificial flavors and sweeteners added. Magnesium citrate capsules are hard to find. If you can't locate them in your neighborhood, you can order them by mail from Hickey Chemists, Ltd., 888 Second Avenue, New York, N.Y. 10017.

Add B Vitamins to Aid Magnesium Absorption. The B vitamins, especially B-1 and B-6, help the body absorb and use magnesium more efficiently. If magnesium alone doesn't solve colic or behavioral problems, add 10 milligrams a day of *vitamin B-6 only* (B complex usually doesn't work as well) to his diet. Your pharmacist can make up a liquid form, free of additives.

If B-6 seems to have no effect, stop it and try 10 milligrams of B-1 (thiamine) a day, in the same liquid form.

Calcium for Temperament. If magnesium alone doesn't seem to help your baby's behavioral problems, add calcium—100 to 200 milligrams a day in the form of liquid calcium carbonate.

THE FOOD CONNECTION

Because many common problems start with food allergies, you may have to do a little nutritional detective work in the form of food trials to discover the food or foods that started the trouble.

This will be your first step in dealing with diarrhea and constipation, spitting up, coughing and congestion, and one form of severe diaper rash. For colic or behavioral problems it is easier to try magnesium first; if that doesn't work, go on to a food trial.[6] For eczema, start with EFAs as I show you below under The EFA Connection, and then do a food trial.

The Food Trial

If you are breast-feeding, first check your own diet. For five days, stop taking all vitamins or drugs (be sure and check with your doctor before stopping any prescribed medication). Stop eating all possibly allergenic foods: milk, wheat products, corn, soy, eggs, caffeine, spices, green, orange, or red vegetables, all fruit. Eat only such "safe" foods as meat (lamb, beef, veal, or pork), poultry, rice, potatoes, and yellow vegetables such as squash. If there is no change by the end of five days, the problem is not your diet; it's your baby's. (The "safe" foods have all been statistically proved to be less allergenic.)

The most common allergen is cow's milk; if you are using a cow's milk formula, try changing to one based on soy. (Casein in the milk could also be causing him to spit up.) If a soy formula doesn't stop the symptom, switch to a formula based on hydrolyzed vegetable protein, such as Nutramigen.

If he is eating solid foods, cut him back to the safe foods, too: rice cereal, lamb, applesauce, and yellow vegetables. If he is taking vitamins, stop them altogether during this period. If his symptoms don't stop after five days, cut out the applesauce and yellow vegetables and feed him only lamb, rice, and breast milk or hydrolyzed formula for five more days.

Once he stops showing symptoms, you can begin to add new foods carefully—one every two days. Feed each new food two or three times a day for two days. Watch carefully to see whether he develops any symptoms; if he does, cut that food out of his diet altogether and go on to the next. You can treat vitamins as you would a food, and add in one at a time.

Food Allergy–Caused Diaper Rash

What looks like diaper rash could be caused by food allergy. If so, the rash comes on suddenly and is bright red—the skin looks scalded. (Both these factors distinguish this rash from that caused by a yeast infection, described below under The Yeast Connection.) Suspect a food eaten by one of you in the last forty-eight hours. It could take another forty-eight hours to clear up, depending on how quickly his body eliminates the toxic material. Because almost any food or additive could be the culprit, I suggest a food trial.

THE STRESS CONNECTION

You might also pay special attention to your own emotional state. Are you under stress? If you are emotionally upset, how do you react? By eating? By not eating? Do you become constipated? Whether or not you are breast-feeding, your behavior and emotional state can trigger changes in your baby's behavior—and that, in turn, can trigger more emotional stress in you.

THE EFA CONNECTION

Diarrhea and Constipation

Since both these conditions may be caused by an allergy, conduct a food trial first. If you don't discover the culprit, then you might suspect an EFA deficiency. (A diet too low in fats can cause diarrhea, too.)

If your baby isn't getting flaxseed oil either directly or in your breast milk, add flaxseed oil to your diet or his. If he is getting flaxseed oil now, give him a larger dose: 1 tablespoon a day. (See pp. 67–68 for suggestions on how to give flaxseed oil to a baby.) You may substitute 1 teaspoon of cod-liver oil or 2 tablespoons of walnut oil for 1 tablespoon of flaxseed oil.

Jeremy's family had a history of heart disease, which led his mother to give him no fats. He was eating solid foods and getting only skim milk when I first saw him at the age of ten months. He was suffering from loose bowel movements. I put him on whole milk and flaxseed oil, to provide both fats and EFAs. Jeremy's diarrhea stopped, and his dry skin became smoother.

Behavioral Problems

When you've tried magnesium and, if necessary, done a food trial, it's time to look at EFAs. If your baby isn't getting flaxseed oil either directly or in your breast milk, add flaxseed oil to your diet or his. If he is getting flaxseed oil now, double the dose for you or for him. You may substitute walnut or cod-liver oil in the following ratios: 1 teaspoon of cod-liver oil for 1 tablespoon of flaxseed oil or 2 tablespoons of walnut oil for 1 tablespoon of flaxseed oil.

If you're not happy with the effects of flaxseed oil, apply 2 capsules of evening primrose or black currant oil directly to his skin each day. (See p. 19 for detailed information on evening primrose oil.)

I've seen these oils improve sleep and temperament in two days to two weeks. Take Jessie—at ten months, she was restless and difficult. It was impossible to hold and cuddle her; she would cry loudly until her face turned red, and she never slept more than two hours at a time. I first changed her from a milk to a soy-based formula. She stopped crying and passing gas, but she continued to be irritable and to sleep badly. Her parents wondered why she was thirsty all the time.

Excessive thirst suggested an EFA problem, but 2 teaspoons of flaxseed oil a day seemed to have no effect. I recommended two capsules of evening primrose oil every day, rubbed into Jessie's skin. Within three days she was no longer thirsty, and was sleeping longer and more soundly. But she was still restless and moved stiffly, so I recommended ¼ ounce of magnesium citrate a day. After two weeks, she was much calmer and moved more easily.

Persistent behavioral problems. If the food trials, magnesium, and EFA supplementation outlined above don't result in significant improvement in your child's "difficult" behavior, and if he has most of the symptoms listed on page 83, it may be time to consult your pediatrician. Dr. Turecki, in his book, *The Difficult Child,* suggests some excellent behavioral stratagems.

Eczema

Some children need more EFAs than others because their bodies don't metabolize EFAs well. Children with eczema have difficulty converting linoleic acid, the major omega-6 EFA, to GLA.[7] Evening primrose oil and black currant oil, which contain GLA, get around this problem.

Such children may also need more omega-3 EFAs; up to 1

tablespoon of flaxseed oil a day by age one may help. Or you may substitute up to 1 teaspoon of cod-liver oil or up to 2 tablespoons of walnut oil. If you are breast-feeding, add EFAs to your own diet.

Food allergy usually complicates eczema, so a food trial of the kind outlined on page 86 could help as well.[8]

At three months, Christopher had severe eczema. His mother, who breast-fed him, was eating a lot of eggs. When she cut them out of her diet, Christopher's condition improved but didn't disappear entirely. To increase omega-3 EFAs in her milk, his mother added flaxseed and cod-liver oil to her diet. Over the next two months Christopher's eczema cleared up and his dry skin improved.

Jennifer at nine months was skinny and a picky eater. Although she had dry skin and mild eczema, I didn't want to start eliminating foods from her diet because she was so thin. Instead, I advised rubbing two primrose oil capsules and 1 teaspoon of flaxseed oil into her skin each day. Her eczema cleared up completely.

SEVERE DIAPER RASH: THE YEAST CONNECTION

Ordinary diaper rash, a light reddening of the skin, can easily be avoided. It's caused by urine and stool, both of which irritate skin. It can be prevented by frequent changes, gentle but thorough cleansing, powdering with cornstarch, and paper diapers, especially in hot weather. If you are breast-feeding your child, he is less likely to get diaper rash, because his stool and urine contain fewer irritating substances than they would if he drank formula.

Severe diaper rash, a persistent angry redness of the skin, is usually a symptom of a yeast infection. The yeast *Candida albicans* thrives in a warm, dark, moist environment, so one step toward a cure is to use powder or let your baby go without a diaper for a while. Desitin, a common over-the-counter cream for diaper rash, contains undecylenic acid, a natural, nonessential fatty acid that inhibits yeast growth and is soothing to the skin. Vitamin A & D ointment stimulates local immune response and is also soothing.

If none of these treatments works, pediatricians sometimes

need to prescribe Mycolog cream, a mixture of cortisone (to decrease inflammation), an antibiotic, and Nystatin (to kill yeast).

To prevent a yeast infection, avoid unneeded antibiotics, whether he gets them through your milk or directly. Antibiotics can make your baby prone to yeast infections,

- If your baby is taking formula, supplement it with *Lactobacillus bifidus* while taking antibiotics. Use either:

  Lactopriv B (soy-based):   3 teaspoons a day
  Bifido-Factor (milk-based):   ½ teaspoon three times a day

  (Both can be found in health-food stores.)

- Keep sugar out of your diet and his, and take flaxseed oil: 1 teaspoon a day for him, 1 tablespoon a day for you.
- Provide a diet rich in zinc, iron, and vitamin A. Egg yolks and liver are the best choices for your baby. Combine them with fruits with a high vitamin C content such as strawberries or oranges, or vegetables such as broccoli or tomatoes. Feed him one egg yolk or 2 ounces of liver every day for two weeks, then reduce the amount to three egg yolks and 2 ounces of liver a week. Don't give him more than that; with too much liver, you risk an overdose of vitamin A.
- Give him Nystatin oral suspension, 500,000 units four times a day before eating for two to four weeks. Nystatin is the only prescription drug I advocate using more aggressively with infants and young children. The widespread and generally excessive use of antibiotics in this country promotes intestinal *Candida* overgrowth, an important factor in promoting allergy. Commonly used doses of Nystatin are often inadequate to reduce this growth; for an infant, 500,000 units will.
- Apply Mycostatin (a form of Nystatin) cream directly to the rash. Aloe vera gel is an effective alternative.

Thrush. This is a painful mouth infection caused by an overgrowth of yeast. The symptoms—white patches adhering to the mucous lining of his mouth, tongue, or throat—may look like tonsillitis. Your pediatrician can make an accurate diagnosis from a throat or white-patch culture.

Nystatin, the antiyeast drug, is routinely prescribed for

thrush. I recommend following the same general course of treatment I outlined above for diaper rash. (Nystatin is a prescription drug; you will need your pediatrician's cooperation.)

RECURRENT INFECTIONS

Recurrent Ear Infections

These are usually caused by allergy-inflamed tissue. Swollen tissue prevents fluid from draining out of the middle ear, and this dammed-up fluid becomes a breeding ground for bacteria. I usually see children with this problem when they are four to eight years old, after they've had multiple infections and their doctors have recommended using tubes to drain the fluid and reduce swelling. In my experience, the real problem is that these children are allergy prone and are not receiving the EFAs—especially omega-3—they need to keep their immune system in good shape. In addition, the antibiotics administered to combat the infection have killed off their normal intestinal bacteria, making room for an overgrowth of yeast. Often a child becomes allergic to *Candida*, leading to respiratory congestion that is usually misdiagnosed as a cold. Treatment varies with age. For infants under one year, I recommend the following:

- Avoid antibiotics unless a bacterial infection is found. Bacterial infections—strep throat, bronchitis, pneumonia, and middle-ear infection—usually cause fever, pain, or shortness of breath. Antibiotics are effective against bacteria, but most colds, sore throats, and coughs are caused by viruses, which do not respond to antibiotics.
- If your child does have a bacterial infection and takes antibiotics, give him 500,000 units of Nystatin (Mycostatin R) suspension four times a day, continuing for a week after he's off the antibiotic. Mycostatin does nothing but kill yeast. If your child has had antibiotics and now has allergic problems, I recommend one additional month of Nystatin treatment.
- Give him *Lactobacillus bifidus* to restore his normal intestinal bacteria.
- Temporarily cut all remaining sugar out of his diet, including fruits and fruit juices. If he is on a cow's milk formula, switch

to soy. Eliminate all other cow's milk–based foods such as yogurt. Once his congestion clears up, you can reintroduce these foods to see which ones he can tolerate.

• Give him 1 to 2 teaspoons of flaxseed oil a day or 2 to 4 teaspoons of walnut oil.

• Give him 500 to 1,000 milligrams of vitamin C a day. In high doses, vitamin C is antiallergenic. If he gets diarrhea, cut back his dosage.

• Make sure his diet is rich in zinc, iron, and vitamin A. We get most vitamin A in the form of carotene, the orange pigment in carrots, and many green, red, and yellow vegetables. Carotene is an excellent antioxidant, but to stimulate the immune system it has to be converted to retinol, or true vitamin A. I have found that many children with recurrent infections seem to have problems making this conversion. They need to eat foods that contain retinol. Good sources are egg yolks and liver, combined with vitamin C to enhance iron absorption. Feed them daily for a month, then cut back to twice a week so you don't overdose your baby with vitamin A.

Cod-liver oil is a good source of both vitamin A and omega-3s, but to avoid a vitamin A overdose, don't give it to your baby if he is also eating liver.

Alexi was a child whose problems started with ear infections. He had been formula fed, and did well until, at six months, he had one or two ear infections and was given antibiotics. After these treatments, he began spitting up hard globs of mucus three or four times a day. When I saw him, at eleven months, he was irritable and cranky. He was eating jarred baby foods and had become very constipated. I switched him from milk to soy formula, and his condition improved. When his mother cut out commercial baby food and puréed his vegetables herself, his spitting up decreased by 90 percent. When he was put back on commercial foods, it returned.

I decided that the antibiotics might have started his problem by killing the "good" bacteria in his intestine and allowing a yeast overgrowth. That, in turn, had probably contributed to a food allergy. I recommended a *Lactobacillus bifidus* supplement (Lactopriv B, a soy-based powder) and a short course of Nystatin to kill the yeast. Alexi's whole problem cleared up.

Excess Mucus, Coughing, Congestion

First, make sure there are no smokers in the house. Then, if you've done a food trial, give your baby the EFAs—especially omega-3—that he probably lacks. One to 2 teaspoons a day of flaxseed oil or 1 tablespoon of walnut oil or cod-liver oil should do it.

In addition, follow the recommendations for supplements detailed above under Recurrent Ear Infections. Mucus, coughing, and congestion can easily turn into a respiratory or ear infection.

Recurrent Respiratory Infections

These may also originate in allergic symptoms and can be treated in the same way as recurrent ear infections.

Nothing can compare with the first year of your child's life, but now he is about to become a toddler. Nothing will compare with this, either: he's about to start showing you that he's an individual with a mind of his own. The next two chapters will deal with this remarkable period.

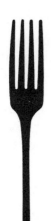

Ages One to Five:
The Supernourished Toddler

Toddlers can be ornery. This is the age when the word *no* enters their vocabulary, and they love to use it. It's perfectly natural. Toddlers are beginning to assert their individuality, their sense of being a separate self, and saying no is their way of setting boundaries.

As a smart mother, you will learn how to outflank, rather than confront, your toddler over getting dressed, going to bed, and all the daily occasions in between. Good strategies are especially important when it comes to food, because if an all-out nutrition war is hard on you, it can be disastrous for your child's eating habits later in life.

There is one basic principle to remember when your toddler says no to food: *You control* what *she eats, and she controls* how much *she eats.* In practice, this means it is not productive to tell a toddler, say, that she won't get cookies unless she eats everything on her plate. It may be tempting to say this when she refuses to eat her carrots, but if you give way to the temptation the end result will be that she will think cookies are one of the most important things in life, while eating carrots is pure punishment.

A good way to look at this problem is that dessert is on the menu, and so are vegetables, or soup, or whatever. You decide the menu, and serve your toddler everything on it. She doesn't get to ask for something that's not on the menu. But if she really can't stand carrots that night, she can decide not to eat them. She will still get dessert, because it's on the menu. And the chances are that if eating carrots has not been made into a sore point, the next time you serve them she will eat them with gusto. (It's a good idea to serve your toddler at the dinner table with the rest of the family, so she can learn that meals are sociable occasions, and that lots of other people actually *like* carrots.)

Another way to deal with this problem—which partly results from the fact that children, like all of us, naturally like sweets—is to make desserts as nutritious as possible, so that when your toddler eats them she is not just consuming sugars and nonessential fats, both of which can weaken her immune system. You will find plenty of home-tested, nutritious dessert recipes in Chapter 10.

Your toddler's immune system is growing up along with her, and this means she will get infections—colds, sore throats, flu, earache. This sounds contradictory, because I have been promising that the nutritional guidelines you are following will bolster your child's defenses. And they will. But you may recall that in Chapter 1 I pointed out that a child's immune system has to be educated. The lymphocytes, those crucial white blood cells that send your child's other defensive cells into action, have to learn to recognize the thousands of germs, viruses, fungi, and other microbes that invade everyone's body in the course of a lifetime.

Each infection your child gets now will serve to teach and strengthen her immune system, so that the next time that microbe invades, she won't get sick. The healthier her lymphocytes are, the faster they will learn—and the more quickly they will call out the cells that destroy invaders. With good nutrition and a well-regulated immune system, most of your toddler's infections should be relatively mild. So one of your jobs is to keep her white blood cells healthy by providing foods rich in EFAs and the key co-factor nutrients that help her body metabolize them. The end result of EFA metabolism is the prostaglandins that keep your child's defense system humming.

You will also want to give your child a good supply of foods containing the antioxidants that fight the damage done to EFAs by free radicals, the "sparks" given off when her body burns pollutants. And, of course, as much as possible you will want to keep anti-nutrients like sugar, partially hydrogenated fats, sodium, and added phosphates out of your child's diet altogether. Anti-nutrients keep her body from metabolizing EFAs, so they are destructive to her immune system. (If you want to refresh your memory on all this, just reread Chapter 1.)

These preschool years are the last time you will have almost complete control over your child's diet. Once she starts going to school, and peer pressure becomes important to her, the temptations of junk foods will become very strong. But at this age she is developing her tastes, and by feeding her nutritious foods that are naturally sweet, for example, you will help her develop a taste for them, rather than the sugar-loaded, too-sweet candies and pastries she will inevitably encounter later on. (Contrary to popular mythology, well-nourished toddlers do not crave sweets, and will normally not stuff themselves with candy or ice cream. A psychologically conditioned craving for sweets is often developed later.) A palate formed on low-salt cooking will find most manufactured foods too salty, and a child who has grown up eating grilled, baked, broiled, or stir-fried fish and poultry may find fast-food hamburgers, chicken nuggets, and deep-fried fish too greasy.

The biggest nutritional challenge facing you now is how to make sure your child gets enough of the important co-factor minerals and vitamins and the antioxidants, as well as certain other key nutrients. Your biggest concerns will be calcium, magnesium, iron, zinc, and vitamin A—in one or several of which far too many toddlers are deficient. The solution is not as simple as, say, drinking a lot of milk to get calcium. As we shall see, this habit, one Americans have traditionally encouraged their children to develop, does not, in fact, make good nutritional sense. But first, as always, we need to look at those crucial EFAs.

KEEPING UP WITH THE EFAs

Your first concern in helping to bolster your child's immune system will be to maintain her supply of EFAs, especially the omega-3s in which most American children are commonly deficient. If you haven't already, you should add flaxseed oil to her diet at this point, in the following doses depending on her age:

> one to two years—1 teaspoon a day
> two to three years—2 teaspoons a day
> three and up—1 tablespoon a day

If flaxseed oil is unavailable, use twice the dosage of walnut oil or half the dosage of cod-liver oil. If your child's skin and hair have become dry and dull, these amounts of flaxseed oil should do the trick. If both hair and skin don't soon regain their natural luster, you can double the doses. Many toddlers can swallow a tablespoon of flaxseed oil like medicine, if it is followed immediately by food or juice. You can mix flaxseed oil into juice (stir well and have her drink it quickly, before the oil and juice separate). Or, you can use flaxseed or walnut oil in dressings, spreads, and for baking. (See pp. 17–18 for ideas, and Chapter 10 for recipes.)

If your child's skin and hair don't improve after this trial, the chances are she needs omega-6 EFAs. Stop the oil you are using and give her an equivalent dose of cold-pressed safflower oil instead. (Safflower oil, too, can be used in dressings, spreads, and for baking.)

BEYOND FLAXSEED OIL

At this age, you can begin to introduce your child to other sources of omega-3 EFAs—*walnut butter* is sometimes hard to find, but it makes a fine substitute for peanut butter. The oil in peanuts is unsaturated, but because of the way the fatty acids are arranged, it promotes cholesterol accumulation—one reason I don't recommend peanut oil for cooking. And commercial brands of peanut butter are often partially hydrogenated. Partial hydrogenation, you will recall, makes perfectly good oils poison to your child's immune system by interfering with the metabolism of EFAs. *Walnuts* can be ground and used as a garnish, as can *flaxseed*.

Now is the time, too, to introduce your toddler to fish, so rich in EFAs. Serve cooked, soft, moist fish twice a week. Start with

such bland fish as cod and haddock—you can slowly encourage
your youngster to try the stronger, more oily, EFA-rich fish such
as tuna and salmon. Avoid freshwater fish and shoreline bottom-
feeders such as flounder and sole because of possible PCB accumulation.

If you are worried about mercury contamination of fish, let
me reassure you. Studies show that mercury levels in salmon have
stayed constant over the years. Whatever amounts of mercury
are found in these deep-water ocean fish occur naturally.

Fresh tuna is far superior to canned, which has had some of
its EFAs removed or destroyed in processing. Look for fish that
is dark rose in color and has a moist surface. If it looks and feels
dry, or is bleached white, or its flesh is separating into segments,
the tuna is no longer fresh—pass it by.

Don't forget another excellent source of EFAs: *beans,* especially soy, kidney, and navy. Beans and *tofu,* made from soybeans, are quadruple values, because they supply protein, minerals, and calcium, too. If you are just becoming acquainted with the
wonderfully versatile tofu, you should know that there are two
kinds: hard and soft. Hard tofu, sold in bricks at many vegetable
markets, has the consistency of a moderately firm cheese. You can
cut it into chunks and broil or stir-fry it, or simmer it in a soup or
stew. Soft tofu has the consistency of a creamy yogurt and can
be used in all the same ways as yogurt, in spreads, toppings, and
shakes, or mixed with fruit. Since tofu has no taste, it will accept
almost any flavor and can be used with any kind of sauce. (See
recipes in Chapter 10.)

Stay away from Tofutti. This ice-cream substitute is ad-
vertised as no-cholesterol, nondairy, and low-calorie, but there
is a big catch: it is loaded with sugar, one of the worst anti-
nutrients.

A RUNDOWN ON ANTIOXIDANTS

No one who eats food can avoid eating pollutants. Chemical toxins
in foods are a major public-health problem today. No food is immune: Grains, nuts, seeds, fruits, and vegetables, unless organically grown, are treated with pesticides. "Factory-raised" chickens, like nonorganically raised cattle, are treated with hormones

and antibiotics and eat feed treated with pesticides and preservatives. Most seafood contains mercury. Even mother's milk contains PCBs.

Your child's antioxidant defense system works to protect her body from damage caused by such environmental pollutants in foods. It also protects her white blood cells from damage in the performance of their duties, and prevents damage to EFAs from the free radicals generated when her cells burn off pollutants.

To do its job, the antioxidant defense system needs particular vitamins—A, C, E, B-2, B-3—and minerals—zinc, copper, manganese, sulfur, and selenium. Your child will need a diet rich in antioxidants all her life; now is a good time to start her on them.

The best food sources of antioxidants are

Vitamin A: carrots, sweet potatoes, winter squash, red peppers, pumpkin, broccoli, and liver

Vitamin C: citrus fruits, tomatoes, strawberries, red peppers, and broccoli

Vitamin E: oatmeal, sunflower seeds, hazelnuts, almonds, and unrefined EFA-rich oils

Vitamin B-2: dairy products

Vitamin B-3: whole grains (except corn)

Zinc: liver, other meat, oysters, and clams

Copper: fish, sesame seeds, tofu, and kidney beans

Manganese: brown rice, oatmeal, split peas, almonds, peanuts, hazelnuts, pecans, walnuts, and blackberries

Selenium: fish, shellfish, and oatmeal

Sulfur: fish and other protein-rich foods, including meat and eggs

A Note on Liver. Some parents have expressed concern about liver in the diet because they've heard that this organ concentrates the toxins, hormones, and antibiotics to which an animal is exposed in its lifetime. It is true that the liver, an organ whose function is to remove toxic substances from the body, will contain pollutants. But liver is an important source of zinc, vitamin A, and other antioxidants as well as iron, and in my experience its nutritional value far outweighs the dangers of any toxins it contains. The best source of liver is cattle raised under "organic" conditions—range grazed, with no feed laced with hormones or antibiotics. Some supermarkets now carry one or more brands of organic beef and liver (Grand Union is one chain that does).

THE MIGHTY MINERALS

THE CALCIUM CONNECTION

Your child is going to need lots of calcium in these years as her bones grow and she uses her legs more and more to walk, run, and climb. She will need about 600 to 800 milligrams a day.

Dairy products are the best source of calcium, but believe it or not, *it is possible to drink too much milk or eat too much yogurt.* Milk and yogurt are very poor in iron and zinc, and in large quantities they will replace in your child's diet foods that supply those essential nutrients. What's more, calcium blocks zinc and iron absorption. The result of too much milk or milk product in the diet is usually iron or zinc deficiency. A total of 16 ounces of dairy products—milk, yogurt, or cottage cheese—each day is plenty. Although yogurt is preferred because it contains *Lactobacillus acidophilus,* I wouldn't insist that a child eat yogurt instead of drinking milk if she prefers milk.

Enough milk or yogurt is important, and I feel that unless your child has a specific intolerance or is allergic to milk, she should have milk products. It is hard to get enough calcium into her if you remove the best sources. Besides, milk provides protein and vitamin A, an important co-factor nutrient in metabolizing EFAs. Whole milk is a source of omega-6 EFAs.

Good nondairy sources of calcium are beans (don't forget tofu) and almonds. Your child might enjoy bean soup, split-pea soup, chili with beans, bean salads, and tortillas, which are made with calcium-rich lime. Chick-peas make a good snack.

Dark green leafy vegetables such as spinach, broccoli, kale, and parsley contain calcium, too, but they also contain oxalic acid, which may interfere with calcium absorption. I don't recommend dark green vegetables as a source of calcium at this age. Broccoli and kale provide vitamins A and C, though, and are worth eating for that reason. If your child has a problem with the relatively bitter taste of dark green leafy vegetables, try steaming broccoli florets *very* briefly (1 to 2 minutes) and serving them with a tahini or tofu dip. This will both enhance their flavor and make them a finger food, much more fun to eat.

Because some nutritionists advise against the use of cow's milk, I have composed the following list. It will show you how hard it is to give a child 600 milligrams of calcium a day without including 16 ounces of milk or yogurt in the diet:

CALCIUM SOURCES

FOOD	QUANTITY	CALCIUM (mg)
Milk	1 cup	288
Yogurt	1 cup	174
Collard greens, cooked	½ cup	152
Dandelion greens, cooked	½ cup	140
Tofu	½ cup	128
Chives, chopped	1 Tb	120
Kale, cooked	½ cup	105
Spinach, cooked	½ cup	83
Chicory greens, cooked	¼ cup	81
Chick-peas, cooked	3 oz	75
Cottage cheese	½ cup	70
Parmesan cheese	1 Tb	69
Chard, cooked	½ cup	65
Broccoli, raw	½ cup	55
Almond butter	1 oz	43
Tortilla	1	42
Cabbage, cooked	¼ cup	41
Bean soup (homemade)	½ cup	41

Should Your Child Take a Calcium Supplement? If she doesn't consume 16 ounces of dairy foods or their equivalent every day, your child will do well to take one. She'll tolerate calcium carbonate supplements nicely in liquid or chewable form. Although I don't recommend this form for adult women, children usually have enough stomach acid to absorb it if it's given with food.

Calcium carbonate is usually derived from ground oyster shells—check the label, and avoid calcium from bone meal or dolomite, which may be contaminated with lead and other toxic metals.[1]

Don't overdo the amount you give your child—too much may interfere with her body's ability to absorb magnesium, iron, and zinc. If she consumes no milk, yogurt, or cheese, 600 milligrams a day of supplemental calcium is plenty, unless she has one of the rare diseases that involves calcium metabolism. Give her the supplements with meals to enhance their absorption.

MAGNESIUM

At this stage, your growing child needs about 5 milligrams of magnesium per pound of body weight, or about 100 to 250 milligrams a day. Magnesium is an important co-factor mineral in the metabolism of EFAs, and a deficiency can contribute to the severity of allergies. So you will want to help your toddler develop a taste for magnesium-rich foods: nuts, seeds, grains such as oats and buckwheat (although buckwheat, technically, is not a true grain), beans (cooked and in salads), tofu, fish, and nut butters (unsalted, with no sugar added). Skip peanut butter or limit it to once a week—it can raise cholesterol levels and interfere with your child's EFA metabolism. Give her almond or walnut butter instead.

Tofu is an excellent meat substitute as well as providing magnesium and calcium.

IRON AND ZINC: TWO FOR THE WHITE BLOOD CELLS

Iron. This is a critical nutrient for toddlers, who need it for the production of the white blood cells that make up their immune system's army, as well as for the red blood cells that carry oxygen in their blood. Ironically, children who drink lots of milk can easily become iron-deficient, because milk contains very little iron and because calcium can block their body's ability to absorb iron from other foods.

Clams and oysters are excellent sources of iron and zinc, but they are shoreline feeders and so, unlike deep-water ocean fish, may contain pollutants. *Never serve them raw.* Chop them up and cook them in a stew.

The best animal source of iron is liver (see p. 99 about liver). Any danger to the toddler from too much vitamin A can be eliminated by limiting liver to no more than 4 ounces a week, unless under a physician's direction.

Sesame butter (tahini) and sunflower meal contain significant amounts of iron, but the body doesn't digest iron from vegetable sources very well. Vitamin C enhances absorption, so serve tahini or sunflower meal in a dip or sauce with broccoli or sweet red peppers. Sunflower seeds could accompany oranges, grapefruit, strawberries, or tomatoes.

Raisins are a good source of iron, but they are also a good

source of tooth decay because they stick to the teeth. Children should brush their teeth after eating any dried fruit (as well as after every meal).

As you will see from the list that follows, it's not easy for a child to meet his need for iron, so iron-poor junk foods have no place in a toddler's diet—food must supply much more than calories.

IRON SOURCES

FOOD	QUANTITY	IRON (mg)
Meats, cooked	2 oz	
Liver		6
Beef		2
Pork		2
Lamb		2
Poultry		1
Shellfish	2 oz	
Oysters, cooked		10
Clams, cooked		3
Fish, cooked	2 oz	1
Seeds		
Sunflower meal	1 Tb	1
Sesame butter	1 Tb	1
Egg yolk	1	1
Blackstrap molasses	1 Tb	3
Raisins	⅓ cup	1
Oats	½ cup	¾

Zinc. This mineral promotes the growth and development of your child's white blood cells, especially the lymphocytes, those T- and B-cells that identify invading germs and send out antibodies to zap the invaders. Zinc also helps keep the thymus gland healthy and productive. This gland is where T- (for thymus) cells are produced and receive their basic training. What's more, zinc plays key roles in overall growth and in the development of the brain. Unfortunately, many children don't get enough of this vital mineral.

The all-time best source of zinc is Atlantic oysters—your toddler needs about 10 milligrams a day, and 1 ounce of Atlantic oysters will give him over 20 milligrams. No other source comes close. But cooked clams, beef, nuts, and seeds such as sesame and pumpkin contain some zinc.

The following list shows the best food sources of zinc.

ZINC SOURCES

FOOD	AMOUNT	ZINC (mg)
Animal		
Crabmeat, steamed	1 oz	1.2
Beef liver	1 oz	1.0
Egg	1	1.0
Beef, ground	1 oz	0.9
Turkey (dark)	1 oz	0.9
Chicken (dark)	1 oz	0.5
Turkey (light)	1 oz	0.4
Chicken (light)	1 oz	0.2
Fish, moist	1 oz	0.2
Vegetable		
Pumpkin seeds	¼ cup	2.0
Sunflower seeds	¼ cup	1.8
Peanuts	¼ cup	1.7
Almonds, filberts	¼ cup	1.0
Molasses	1 Tb	0.9
Black-eyed peas, cooked	¼ cup	0.8
Mango	half	0.7
Walnuts, pecans	¼ cup	0.6
White beans, cooked	¼ cup	0.5

To get 10 milligrams of zinc a day, a toddler might eat these foods:

FOOD	ZINC (mg)
3 oz dark turkey	3.6
2 Tb almond butter	1.0
¼ cup black-eyed peas	0.8
½ cup oatmeal	0.6
2 slices whole wheat bread	1.2
½ cup brown rice	1.8
¼ cup peas	0.4
½ cup carrots	0.3
¼ cup lima beans	0.1
Total	*9.8*

Your toddler can get half of what she needs from such unrefined, low-zinc foods as fish, brown rice, vegetables, and beans; the other half should come from such high-zinc foods as poultry, nuts, seeds, eggs, and meat. A seafood stew containing minced oysters (see recipes in Chapter 10) served once a week will give a zinc boost to her diet.

Although wheat bran contains zinc, the phytate in the bran blocks its absorption, which is why I don't advocate it for toddlers. *I also don't advocate zinc supplementation,* except under medical supervision. At any age too much zinc will block iron and selenium uptake and lower body levels of copper and manganese, two other vital minerals.

Studies of children with recurrent infections show that they have lower blood levels of iron and zinc than do healthy children. These low levels persist even between the children's bouts with infection, suggesting that zinc and iron deficiencies may cause susceptibility to infection.[2] This is what happened to Joshua.

Joshua was three years old when I saw him. He seemed to catch everything that was going around—colds, diarrhea, bronchitis. If someone in the neighborhood had an infection, Josh caught it. He'd be sick for a week or two, then recover. Fortunately, his pediatrician was not big on antibiotics, which can do harm to young children. (And could not have done any good against his infections, anyway, since they were all virus based.)

When I examined Josh, he was between infections and seemed to be a healthy, active toddler with no evidence of allergies. He didn't eat a lot of sugar, and his parents, who knew something about nutrition, served him few red meats. Josh liked milk, and got about half his calories from whole milk, yogurt, and cottage cheese. He certainly didn't seem to be allergic to milk, but his diet was clearly low in zinc and iron. Sure enough, I found white spots on his fingernails, a sign of zinc—and sometimes of iron—deficiency. Josh wasn't anemic, but a blood test showed that he had a low level of ferritin, the protein that stores iron in the body.

To confirm a zinc deficiency, we analyzed a sample of Josh's hair. (Hair mineral analysis has become controversial because of abuse by irresponsible practitioners, but it is a proven method for assessing zinc status. It is also relatively inexpensive, and it is far less traumatic to a toddler to snip a few hairs from his head than it is to draw blood.) Josh's hair zinc was quite low.

Liver and red meat are good sources of both iron and zinc, but Josh's parents did not want to serve more of them. To encourage him to eat a wider variety of foods, I advised his parents to limit his total consumption of milk, yogurt, and cottage cheese to 16 ounces a day. Then I put him on liquid iron and zinc supplements. He took these for four months, at meal times, until the spots disappeared from his nails.

At that point, we reanalyzed Josh's diet. His parents had been using sunflower meal in his cereal, serving seafood stew once a week, and giving him more fish and poultry. Together with less milk, this regimen had significantly raised the amounts of zinc and iron in his diet, and I took him off the supplements.

After two more months, Josh's immune system had grown much stronger and more active. His infections became milder, shorter, and, finally, fewer. He even escaped a few epidemics that swept his neighborhood.

Why not continue the zinc and iron supplements indefinitely? Because while children need the *right* amount of iron and zinc, too much can be harmful. Population studies show that high iron and zinc levels are associated with increased risk of cancer in adulthood. Experimental studies with animals suggest a method by which this could work: too much zinc may induce cancer by depleting the body's levels of manganese and selenium. Excess iron also lowers manganese levels.

Good nutrition derives from a balance, not megadoses, of nutrients.

VITAMIN A

Vitamin A serves both as a co-factor nutrient, helping the enzymes in your child's body metabolize EFAs, and as an antioxidant, protecting his white blood cells and other cells from attacks by free radicals and from overheating while killing germs or burning off toxins. It is also crucial to healthy skin and good vision.

A recent study at the National Institutes of Health discovered that a single virus infection (in this case, chicken pox) depletes the vitamin A levels of healthy children for several months.[3]

The RDA for vitamin A is:

> Ages   one to three—2,000 units a day
> four to five—2,500 units a day

The best sources of vitamin A are orange, red, yellow, and deep green vegetables such as carrots, squash, sweet potatoes, and spinach, and red, orange, and yellow fruits such as watermelon and apricots. These all contain carotene, an orange pigment that your child's body metabolizes into retinol, the active form of vitamin A. Since her body controls the rate at which carotene is converted to retinol, and does not make more retinol than she needs, vitamin A from vegetable sources is never toxic.

Animal sources of vitamin A, such as liver, whole milk, and egg yolks, contain retinol, so it is possible for your child to get too much vitamin A from these sources. Even so, while toddlers are more susceptible to vitamin A toxicity than older children, amounts of retinol under 10,000 units a day are not likely to be toxic, even for them.

As the following lists show, it is not hard to give your child foods that contain enough vitamin A for her needs—you just have to know which ones to serve.

RETINOL SOURCES

FOOD	AMOUNT	RETINOL (units)
Egg yolk	1	600
Liver		
beef or calf	1 oz	10,000
chicken	1 oz	3,500
Whole milk	1 cup	350
Cod-liver oil	1 Tb	10,000

CAROTENE SOURCES

FOOD	AMOUNT	CAROTENE (units)
Vegetables		
Sweet potato	1 small	8,100
Pumpkin, cooked	¼ cup	4,000
Carrots, cooked	¼ cup	4,000
Collard greens, cooked	¼ cup	4,000
Carrot, raw	1 small	3,500
Winter squash, cooked	¼ cup	2,100
Spinach, cooked	¼ cup	2,000
Broccoli, cooked	½ cup	1,800
Tomato	1 medium	1,400
Tomato juice	½ cup	800
Fruits		
Mango	1	11,000
Watermelon	8 oz wedge	5,000
Cantaloupe	4 oz wedge	3,400
Apricots (fresh)	1 cup	2,200

SEVEN COMMON QUESTIONS ABOUT FEEDING TODDLERS

The pages that follow will provide some simple, commonsense answers to the questions I am most frequently asked about the general care and feeding of toddlers.

DOES A TODDLER NEED FIBER?

If you are following my nutritional guidelines, you don't need to worry about whether your toddler is getting enough fiber. Toddlers have small stomachs, and high-fiber foods are bulky. If your child eats oats, some beans, and some nut butters, plus a variety of vegetables, he will get all the fiber he needs. Wait until he is older before thinking about giving him such concentrated fiber foods as bran.

WHAT ABOUT VEGETARIAN DIETS?

Some people think that a vegetarian diet is a good way to avoid the fat and toxins in meats. But there are many reports of single and multiple nutritional deficiencies among vegetarian children, most commonly vitamin B-12, zinc, iron, and protein. Frances Moore Lappé's *Diet for a Small Planet* and the companion volume *Recipes for a Small Planet* by Ellen Buchman Ewald focus on combining grains, seeds, nuts, beans, and dairy products in high-protein dishes, but neither book adequately covers other nutrients. (The worst-nourished patients I've seen are casual vegetarians: they avoid animal foods but don't make the effort to include mineral- and protein-rich plant foods.)

Macrobiotic diets are low in toxins because they include a very limited range of foods, but they are also low in nutrients, and can be severely damaging to children unless they include fish and soy products as sources of protein, zinc, iron, and B-12.

WHAT ARE THE BEST SNACKS FOR TODDLERS?

All children like snacks, and in addition to three nutritionally balanced meals each day, an active child will need two or three nutritionally sound snacks. A good way to think about snacks is that they provide a handy way to give your child the nutrients he doesn't get in his regular meals—you can even think of them as "minimeals" that provide a mix of protein, carbohydrates, and fat.

Many parents think a piece of fruit is a perfect snack. It's not. Why? Because an apple or pear won't be enough to keep your child satisfied until the next meal. Milk and yogurt provide the right nutrients and are filling enough to keep the most active child happy until mealtime. Their big plus, of course, is calcium. In fact, snacks are the perfect way to fill a toddler's daily calcium needs. Even though it's liquid, milk is really more a food than a drink, and the toddler who drinks it with meals may find he has little room left for other foods. But as the perfect snack, milk offers protein, EFAs, and vitamin A as well as calcium. Feed milk at snack time, not at meals.

With a glass of milk, you can serve low-sugar oatmeal-sesame cookies, a homemade sugar-free granola bar, or a dried fruit and nut bar (see recipes in Chapter 10). Or try carrot sticks dipped in almond butter, or a whole wheat pita bread pizza. As an alternative to milk mix plain yogurt with fresh or frozen berries and chopped nuts, and serve tofu in a strawberry smoothie (see recipe).

ARE CONVENIENCE FOODS OKAY?

As we saw in Chapter 1, most manufactured foods are loaded with fats, sugar, and/or salt, all anti-nutrients and all destructive to your child's immune system. But these days it's virtually impossible to avoid using some convenience foods, such as cereal and canned foods.

Cereals. Commercial cold cereals, including bran and granola, are usually loaded with sugar and salt, and are often made with partially hydrogenated vegetable oils as well. These are particularly lethal because they contain artificial unsaturated fatty acids that block EFA metabolism. Luckily, it's easy to make a big batch of your own low-sugar granola; my recipe is in Chapter 10.

If you're really pressed for time, some commercial cereals are low in sugar: plain Cheerios, shredded wheat (which contains neither sugar nor added salt), puffed wheat, puffed rice, Uncle Sam, Wheat Chex, Grape-Nuts Flakes, Alpen, sugar-free Familia, Special K, Corn Total, and Nutri-Grain. You don't have to worry about the fiber in these cereals; your healthy toddler can handle it well. Unfortunately, most of these cereals are loaded with salt, containing 150 to 300 milligrams of sodium per ounce. Two ounces a day is not a problem, but if your child eats more cereal, these may significantly raise sodium intake.

Canned Foods. The problem with these is that, in addition to being full of salt and/or sugar, the seams of the cans are soldered with lead, which can leach into the food. It's much better to use foods packed in glass. In any case, *never* store opened canned food in the can. Transfer it to a glass jar and refrigerate. And limit the use of canned items to once a week. Canned meats and fish can be used occasionally, and some vegetables are now being canned without added salt or sugar.

Convenience Health Foods. Watch out for these. As we saw above, commercial granolas are full of partially hydrogenated vegetable oil and often contain sugar and salt. Granola bars are too. Products labeled "light" or "lite" are usually as caloric and full of additives as other manufactured foods—they're just more expensive. In health-food stores, though, you can usually find whole-grain breads and crackers made without preservatives or partially hydrogenated vegetable oils. The Scandinavian crisp breads sold in grocery stores generally contain no added fats or preservatives; check the labels. Kavli or Wasa Lite Rye are best. Whole wheat pita is also good.

Do-It-Yourself Convenience Foods. The best convenience foods are the ones you make yourself, because you'll know exactly what goes into them. You can keep fast foods on hand by "batch-cooking"—cooking up a big batch of food and then storing it in portion-size quantities in the freezer.

CAN YOU TAKE A TODDLER TO McDONALD'S?

Tempting as they are when you're pressed for time, avoid both fast-food places and pizza parlors. Most fast-food places fry or deep-fry their food with partially hydrogenated vegetable oil, a double threat because frying creates the free radicals that damage your child's immune system and other cells. Pizza is all right if you can get the real thing, made with real cheese and fresh tomatoes. But today most pizza is made with imitation cheese and tomato sauce. Imitation cheese is concocted with partially hydrogenated vegetable oil flavored to taste like cheese; imitation tomato sauce is an artifically colored, tomato-flavored chemical soup.

WHAT IF ALL THE PARENTS TAKE THEIR KIDS TO McDONALDS?

There is no question that eating is an important occasion for socializing, and, for toddlers, an important experience in socialization. But for the most part, there is no reason to compromise your high standards of nutrition. You can pack a picnic basket and take it to the park or playground. Your child can meet other children her age and perhaps even ask them to share her snack.

If you visit another home with your youngster and inappropriate foods are served for a meal or snack, you can ask whether something more appropriate could be substituted. If you discuss your child-feeding philosophy with the other adults there, you may find that they agree with you! If you meet some defensiveness, it may come from confusion; with a few minutes' discussion you can probably clarify the situation and hit upon one or more foods your hosts have on hand that will suit your child's needs. Good nutrition isn't difficult; it's simply a matter of making the right choices and declining what's not appropriate. In any case, you never need to defend your methods to another parent. In a pinch, you can simply state that you feed your child in a certain way because you believe it's healthy and nourishing.

Which brings us back to those all but inevitable visits to the local fast-food place. In fact, since you're providing your child with good nutrition every day, it won't hurt her to compromise perhaps once a week by having a slice of pizza or a Big Mac with the other kids. Socialization, after all, is often a matter of compromise. The main thing is that she is eating properly as a matter of habit. Too many other children eat poorly as a matter of habit; for them, fast food is just one more item in an already poor diet.

HOW DO YOU HANDLE A PICKY EATER, OR A CHILD ON A MILK KICK WHO WON'T EAT ANYTHING ELSE?

Toddlers are quirky about food as about many other things, and there's no point in making an issue out of it. Don't threaten or bribe yours or capitulate to requests for changes in the menu. Most of all, don't panic. There's no point in asking your two-year-old what she wants to eat. Just provide the healthy foods she needs, and let her eat as much of them as she wants. She won't starve; eventually, she'll eat.

You can help by serving foods that look good and taste good. Be creative. If she won't drink milk, add milk or yogurt to soup, cereal, fruit pops, or smoothies. If she won't eat vegetables, mash or cream them into soups or stews. If she will only eat soft or sweet foods, you can mash or purée the "sweet" vegetables: yams, carrots, acorn squash, or peas. Or you can mix something sweet and nutritious, such as orange juice, into her food.

If she's partial to salty foods, try mixing something salty but nutritious, such as cheese, into her food. You can flavor foods with such herbs or spices as fresh parsley, cinnamon, nutmeg, or ginger. Almost everything tastes better with a sprinkle of lemon juice.

If you decide to add salt to anything, use sea salt; it not only tastes better, it's better for your child because it's rich in magnesium. Magnesium-enriched salt, sold as "Corrected Salt," available from Multiway Associates, is another choice.

If she only wants to drink milk, you have to limit her to 16 ounces a day; sooner or later, she'll get hungry and eat other things.

A TODDLER MEAL PLAN

Planning meals for toddlers involves some of the same considerations you use in planning meals for adults or older children: you want to serve a variety of foods, including, whenever possible, something your toddler really likes. Serving different-colored foods is an attractive way to get nutritional variety, as though nature had chosen color with this in mind. For instance, try to serve one green and one yellow, orange, or red vegetable at both lunch and supper. If you start your toddler on crisp, crunchy salads and vegetable snacks, he will develop a taste for fresh raw vegetables.

- Give your toddler small quantities of several different foods at each meal. That way, he can ask for more if he particularly likes one thing. He will also feel he has more control over how much he eats.
- Plan desserts as an integral, nutritious part of the meal, not as a junk-food "treat."
- Limit your toddler's intake of added sugar to just 1 teaspoon a day. This includes sugar you or a manufacturer adds as an ingredient in other foods.

A Note About Cooking Utensils and Food Storage

Don't cook with aluminum, especially acid foods such as tomato sauce. You can actually see spaghetti sauce etch the aluminum out of pots. I like cast iron the best for cookware. Well-seasoned cast iron is easy to maintain, cooks evenly, and adds iron to food. Glass (Corning Ware) and porcelain are also nontoxic.

The only nontoxic food wrap is wax paper. Plastic wrap contains potentially carcinogenic plasticizers, and aluminum foil can be toxic unless you line it with wax paper. If you store food in Ziploc plastic bags, wrap it in wax paper first.

The following guidelines will provide your toddler with a

healthful, nutritious diet that will help him develop strong resistance to infections, strong bones, and a lifelong taste for foods that are both delicious and good for him.

FIVE MEALS A DAY

This is a good schedule for *active* toddlers and preschoolers:

> Breakfast
> Midmorning snack
> Lunch
> Midafternoon snack
> Supper

FOODS TO INCLUDE

FOOD	SERVING SIZE	FREQUENCY
Milk or yogurt	2 cups	Daily, no more than this (Limit hard cheese to three 2-oz servings a week.)
Meat	2 oz (a serving size roughly 2 by 2 by ¼ inches)	Once a week
Poultry	2 oz (roughly 2 by 2 by ¼ inches)	Up to three meals a week
Fish	2 oz (roughly 2 by 2 by ¼ inches)	Two meals a week, minimum; more, if possible
Egg	1	One a day
Nut butter	2 Tb	Daily
Beans	½ cup	Two meals a week, at least
Tofu	3 oz	Two meals a week, at least
Fruit (Emphasize fruits high in vitamin C, such as oranges, grapefruit, or berries in season.)	½ cup	Three servings daily

Vegetables (Emphasize those high in vitamins A and C, such as tomatoes, sweet potatoes, and broccoli.)	2 Tb	Six servings daily
Whole-grain bread	½ slice	
Cooked cereal	¼ cup	Three servings daily
Dry cereal	⅓ cup	

BREAKFAST

This should be a high-protein meal. Leftovers from supper would be good, but most Americans don't want fish or beans first thing in the morning. Here are some good high-protein toddler breakfasts:

Cereal: Oatmeal, the all-time favorite, is still the best. Don't add salt. Flavor it with fresh fruit or raisins. Milk is optional; if your child doesn't get enough during the day, add it now. You can flavor oatmeal with cinnamon, sunflower seeds, and raisins to supply magnesium, calcium, zinc, vitamin A, and iron.

Alternatives to oatmeal? Try homemade Swiss muesli (see recipes in Chapter 10) which is sold commercially as sugar-free Familia, with plain yogurt or whole milk and fruit. This supplies calcium, magnesium, and vitamins A and C. You can also serve homemade granola (see Chapter 10) or the commercial cereals listed on page 110.

Egg. Serve one poached or medium-boiled, with whole wheat toast and orange juice. Or serve whole-kernel grits instead of bread. This supplies zinc, iron, and vitamins A and C. As a general rule don't serve fried or scrambled eggs; frying oxidizes the cholesterol, producing toxic by-products that can damage blood vessels.

Since eggs supply protein, iron, and zinc, serve one a day unless your family has a history of cholesterol problems. This means that a close relative—mother, father, grandparent, uncle, or aunt—has had a heart attack before the age of sixty.

Wheat-soy pancakes (see recipe in Chapter 10) can be cooked in batches in advance and frozen. Served with fresh or puréed frozen blueberries, they supply magnesium, calcium, and vitamins A and C.

Sesame Waffles with applesauce (see Chapter 10) supply magnesium and zinc.

Some other breakfast foods:

Bread and crackers. Use only those listing 100 percent whole wheat flour (or other whole grains) as the first ingredient.

Spreads. Nut butters are best. For sweetness, use unsweetened apple butter instead of heavily sugared jams or jellies. A few unsweetened fruit spreads are beginning to appear in supermarkets, but they are expensive. Sorrell Ridge conserves, without sugar or honey, are delicious and worth a try.

Beverages. Orange juice is best; I recommend grapefruit juice, too. Unless they are fortified, other juices are lower in vitamin C. Serve milk only for snacks, not at mealtimes.

LUNCHES AND SNACKS
(Midmorning, Noon, and Midafternoon)

Snack foods and lunch foods are basically interchangeable—in fact, think of lunch as another snack, equal in size to your child's midmorning and midafternoon snacks. If she has had a good breakfast, and if she's likely to eat a family supper, make lunches and snacks light and easy.

Soups. Homemade are best. Canned or dried instant soups usually contain far too much salt and other anti-nutrients. (In a pinch, Goya or Progresso are acceptable.)

Sandwiches. Use whole-grain breads. Use nut and fruit butters. Limit fatty spreads such as mayonnaise to 1 teaspoon a day. (It's best to avoid most commercial mayonnaise altogether. You can get natural mayonnaise, made with soy oil, in health-food stores. Best of all, make your own, with flaxseed or walnut oil. See Chapter 10.)

Leftover meat, poultry, or fish makes an excellent sandwich filling. Stay away from lunch meats such as pressed ham or bologna—they're too high in salt and fat.

Yogurt. Add fresh fruit, chopped nuts, or seeds and flaxseed or walnut oil.

Finger foods. Youngsters love them. Carrot sticks are good plain or dabbed with nut butter, as are zucchini sticks, blanched asparagus tips, and blanched broccoli or cauliflower florets. The last three are especially high in vitamin C, as are peas, three-bean salad, green pepper strips, and tomato wedges.

Don't serve pretzels or potato chips, both of which are too salty and soaked in heat-damaged oils.

A checklist of other possibilities
(See recipes in Chapter 10 for asterisked items):
• Low-salt cottage cheese with fresh fruit
• Nut butter on carrot sticks, or Hummus* on celery
• Homemade Granola Bar*
• Homemade Bean Soup:* cook a batch in advance and freeze in 4-ounce servings
• Tofu crisps (sautéed tofu) with sea salt
• Smoothies:* soft tofu or yogurt puréed with banana or other fresh fruit and nut butter
• Whole-grain crackers or whole wheat pita with nut butter and apple butter, or with cheese (Best crackers are Kavli or Wasa lite rye, no fats added.)
• Tuna or chicken salad prepared with homemade flaxseed or walnut oil Mayonnaise,* served plain, on whole-grain bread
• Mini-pizza made with a Whole Wheat Muffin,* cheese, and to-mato*
• Any breakfast makes a fine lunch or snack; so do leftovers from supper.

SUPPER

Make supper a light meal, too—it ensures a good night's sleep for everyone. Since it's usually the only meal at which the whole family eats together, include your toddler and give her the same foods everyone else eats.

Supper should usually include the following foods:

Starch. Brown rice, baked potato (mash your child's with a little milk, yogurt, or soft tofu), corn, whole-grain bread, or kasha. Kasha is rich in minerals, especially magnesium.

Vegetables. Two, perhaps one green and one orange or yellow, for vitamins A and C. The best way to prepare vegetables is to steam them as briefly as possible to tenderize them. If necessary, mash them for your child. Or you can cut them with a cookie cutter to make interesting shapes. A small amount of grated cheese adds flavor.

Protein. Limit red meat to one serving a week. Despite advertising to the contrary from meat producers, there is too much saturated fat even in lean red meat. Liver is the best choice because it is rich in folic acid and vitamin A, zinc, and iron, all key nutrients for building a strong immune system. (See recipes in Chapter 10 for liver dishes.)

Poultry is a good source of protein and the dark meat is rich in zinc and iron as well. The main problem with poultry is its contamination by hormones, antibiotics, and pesticides. Furthermore, many commercial chickens have cancerous tumors that are removed before they go to the supermarket. They are intrinsically unhealthy birds. They can be legally sold if one tumor was present, but not if two were found. The best birds are raised without hormones, antibiotics, or pesticide-treated grain, and are range-fed. Bell and Evans is a brand sold nationally.

Serve seafood—shellfish or fish—two or three times a week. Seafood is low in saturated fat and high in omega-3 EFAs and important minerals. Stews and soups are tasty ways to serve seafood and are easy to prepare. (See Chapter 10.)

Serve beans at least twice a week. Besides providing protein, they're excellent sources of magnesium, soluble fiber, minerals, and *lectins,* starchy compounds that stimulate the immune cells of the intestine. You can add shredded or grated cheese for tanginess.

Some of the tastiest ways to prepare high-protein foods also provide important nutrients:

Bouillabaisse made with oysters, clams, cod, carrots, peas, tomatoes, potatoes, or rice. Serve at least once a week. (See recipes in Chapter 10.) Rich in EFAs, zinc, iron (shellfish), selenium (fish), vitamin A (carrots and tomatoes), and vitamin C (tomatoes). An excellent immune booster.

Broiled fish almondine with brown rice, lemon, broccoli, tomatoes, and almonds. Provides magnesium, selenium, and vitamins A and C.

Brown rice and pinto beans with sweet red peppers (see Chapter 10). Rich in magnesium and vitamins A and C.

Pasta and white beans with tomato and escarole (see Chapter 10). Supplies magnesium, folic acid, and vitamins A and C.

Roast poultry. Dark meat turkey is the best; it's richest in zinc and iron. (See recipes in Chapter 10 for stuffing.) In the same oven, bake a winter squash or sweet potato to provide vitamins A and C. Steam cauliflower or asparagus tips.

Stir-fried vegetables, such as carrots, broccoli florets, water chestnuts, and Chinese celery and cabbage; add tofu or sliced meat or poultry and bean sprouts (mung or adzuki); serve over white or brown rice. Supplies vitamin A, magnesium, and protein. (*Note:* Young toddlers may have trouble with the crunchy vegetables, but should have no problem with tofu, rice, and sprouts.)

DESSERTS

These are traditional after supper or dinner. They should be a nutritious part of the meal, not a special treat. Don't use desserts as a bribe to get your child to eat other foods; that will just make them seem more important than they really are.

The following desserts are delicious and wholesome.

Homemade freezer pops. Although they are messy, youngsters enjoy them. You can make your own very easily: Buy metal molds, pour in plain juice with puréed or mashed fruit mixed with yogurt, and freeze. Do not add sugar.

Fruit salad. Orange and grapefruit slices for vitamin C, plus other fruits in season. For crunchiness and magnesium, top with chopped nuts. For texture, calcium, and protein top with yogurt or soft tofu.

Fresh fruit in season. Baked apple with cinnamon, natural (unsweetened) applesauce with raisins, berries topped with plain yogurt and chopped nuts, or peaches over cottage cheese with sesame seeds.

Low-sugar pastries made with whole-grain flour and dried fruit: sugar-free oatmeal raisin cookies, apple-coconut muffins, spice cake (see recipes in Chapter 10).

Sugar-free pies with whole-wheat crusts and cooked fresh fruit or fruit-tofu fillings, like pumpkin-tofu pie (see recipes in Chapter 10).

Yogurt sundae. Blend yogurt with banana or berries, top with mixed nuts, cinnamon, or nutmeg. Chill.

Fruit-juice snow cone or frozen fruit juice pops.

Smoothies (see recipes in Chapter 10).

Low-sugar tofu pudding (see recipes in Chapter 10).

These desserts supply nutrients to complement the day's meals. If your child hasn't eaten much yogurt or drunk much milk that day, choose one of the yogurt or tofu recipes. If she hasn't eaten citrus fruits or tomatoes, choose a fruit dessert and include a citrus fruit. If she hasn't gotten much magnesium, choose a tofu- or nut-based recipe.

If you follow this diet plan carefully, your child will eat and drink an ample supply of the nutrients that, at this age, are most important both for growth and for a healthy immune system.

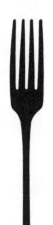

Nutritional First Aid
to Fight Toddler Illnesses

Toddlers are beginning to get out into the world, and inevitably they will come down with illnesses of one kind or another. Their immune systems are still meeting new challenges. Fortunately, most common toddler illnesses—stomachaches, colds, some recurrent bacterial infections, allergies, even chronic behavioral problems—respond very well to nutritional therapy. In fact, in many cases these problems are actually symptoms of nutritional deficits.

If your child has rough, dry skin or hair, is constipated, and/or frequently gets stomachaches, colds, sore throats, or ear infections, he probably has a nutritional problem. If his eyes are puffy or he has dark circles under them, if he has persistent drippy nose or nighttime cough, if he's over four but still constantly wets his bed, or if he has frequent mood changes, he may well have a food allergy.

America as a society relies heavily on drugs, and in some cases, particularly middle-ear infections, drugs are needed to clear up a problem. But drugs, especially antibiotics, can also create their own problems, and those can be most effectively dealt with through nutrition. In other cases, such as colds, reaching for the aspirin or Tylenol is not usually the best course, particularly with a toddler. Nutrition will do a better job. Your child will come out of his illness with a healthier immune system that will probably be able to fight off the next invasion of virus or bacteria.

In the pages that follow I shall give you step-by-step procedures to follow for the most common toddler illnesses. But first, it's useful to know the signs of simple nutritional deficiency.

SIGNS OF A SIMPLE NUTRITIONAL DEFICIENCY

A deficiency in a specific nutrient can announce itself with a single symptom. The cure is simple; refer to Chapter 5 and supply your toddler with the right amount of that nutrient:

SYMPTOM	POSSIBLE DEFICIENCY
Dry or rough skin or hair	EFAs
White spots on nails	Zinc or iron
Constipation	Magnesium or fiber
Craving for sweets	This is a sign not of a single deficiency but of general undernutrition.

Well-fed, well-nourished toddlers don't crave sweets. Conditioned, or psychological, cravings for sugar come later. Toddlers will eat a small amount of ice cream or candy, but they won't stuff themselves. The solution to this problem is to read Chapter 5 and apply the principles of toddler nutrition detailed there to your child.

Still, toddlers are not immune to social pressures, especially TV advertising. So there will be times when your well-fed toddler will badger you for sweets. Don't give in. At home, give him the food *you* want him to eat, but don't force him to eat it. Just leave it out for him; sooner or later, he'll get hungry and eat it. If you're in the supermarket and he spots a sugar-coated cereal or candy he's seen on TV, move to another area. If you're in the checkout line, try to ignore him. Or divert him; change the subject. Point out how interesting the checkout procedure is.

Now, let's look at some common toddler illnesses.

STOMACHACHES

This is the commonest health problem among toddlers. The pain can range from relatively mild to excruciating, but the cure is usually simple. Investigators at McMaster University in Ontario studied digestive complaints in 149 healthy two-year-olds. Constipation was a chronic problem in 16 percent, diarrhea in 8 percent, and abdominal pain in 5 percent. Altogether 27 percent had some kind of chronic intestinal disturbance. By the age of forty months only 5 percent had intestinal problems. The main difference between affected and unaffected youngsters was in fluid consumption. Toddlers with digestive complaints consumed almost twice as much fluid, usually as fruit juice, than toddlers without digestive complaints. The investigators speculated that the high carbohydrate-to-fat ratio of fruit juices may not be tolerated by some toddlers below three years of age. As discussed above, infants and toddlers need relatively more dietary fat than adults. If you follow the diet plan outlined in Chapter 5, your toddler will not experience this problem. If digestive problems occur despite this dietary program, and your child does not drink more than four to five 8-ounce glasses of liquid a day or no more than two glasses of juice, then the cause might well be a calcium or magnesium deficiency. If your child is constipated, give him 1 tablespoon of magnesium citrate each day. If, on the other hand, his bowels are loose, try a calcium-magnesium supplement. Grind up one Bronson Cal-Mag tablet and mix it into applesauce. Give him this twice a day.

Often, the culprit in stomachaches is a food allergy—most often milk. If your child doesn't respond to magnesium, then the nutritional detective work outlined in Chapter 4 will tell you whether this is the case with your toddler.

INFECTIONS

There are two common sources of infection: viruses, which cause colds, flu, measles, mumps, and chicken pox; and bacteria, which cause inflammation, soreness, and other symptoms in a specific part of the body such as the ear or the respiratory tract. Viruses and bacteria are very different, and the ways of treating the infections they cause are different, too. Antibiotics, for example, are useful against ear infections but useless against viral infections such as flu or measles.

COLDS AND OTHER VIRAL INFECTIONS

If your child comes down with any viral infection:
- *Don't force food on him.* Loss of appetite is normal and protective—eating less temporarily boosts the immune response.
- *Prevent dehydration.* Give him liquid every fifteen to thirty minutes. A mouthful every fifteen minutes will do. Orange juice diluted with water is a good choice because it provides some vitamin C.
- *Give him vitamin C.* About 500 milligrams every three hours. If his bowels become loose, stop giving it that day. The next day, give him 200 milligrams every three hours. If his bowels again become loose, stop C that day; the next day, give him 100 milligrams every 4 hours. Then give him about 500 milligrams a day until he's recovered.

Although some claim that megadoses of vitamin C are not utilized by the body and are just excreted in the urine, vitamin C in doses of 1,000 milligrams a day or more has been shown to enhance immune function in normal human volunteers.[1]
- *Give vitamin A.* One tablespoon of cod-liver oil a day for five days. Viral infections produce a depletion of vitamin A stores in the liver that can last for several months.[2] An Australian study of well-nourished children with recurrent respiratory infections found that vitamin A supplementation significantly reduced the frequency of further infection, even though the children had normal blood levels of vitamin A.[3] Allergic children showed the most benefit. Vitamin A as retinol stimulates the killer T-cells in his blood. In addition, cod-liver oil contains omega-3 EFAs that help fight inflammation.
- *If he has liquid diarrhea.* Don't give him more than 200 milligrams of vitamin C a day. Don't give him any cod-liver oil. Diarrhea causes the loss of both water and salt. To replace them, keep him off solid food and give him a mouthful of liquid every five to ten minutes. Dilute one part fruit juice with two parts water and add a pinch of salt; this will supply fluid, sodium, potassium, and sugar, needed by the intestines to combat diarrhea. For potassium and sugar, you can also feed him very

ripe, mashed banana. At this age concern about pesticide residues in bananas becomes secondary to their nutritional value in the treatment of diarrhea.

Once the diarrhea has stopped, give him high-magnesium foods—nuts, kasha, or seafood—or a magnesium supplement for a week or two. Since magnesium itself is a laxative, keep the supplement dosage small—a good choice is liquid magnesium citrate, easily available: 1 teaspoon a day for ten days. This is a sublaxative dose. A four- or five-year-old can manage 1 tablespoon a day.

- *I don't recommend Tylenol or aspirin to control fever* unless a child's temperature is 103° F. or greater, or he is in pain. A slight fever stimulates the immune system, but toddlers can go into convulsions if their fevers rise above 104° F.
- *I'm not impressed with antihistamines and cough medicines.* Hot water or lemon and honey is good for loosening a dry, hacking cough. Vitamin C at the doses I list above is a good decongestant.

BACTERIAL INFECTIONS

Ear Infections

Among toddlers, these are the most common infections. Middle-ear infections need to be treated aggressively with antibiotics to prevent meningitis. Unfortunately, though, antibiotics kill bacteria indiscriminately, including good bacteria in the mouth and intestines. These good bacteria prevent the growth of such undesirable organisms as yeast, which, when it grows unchecked, can have some unpleasant consequences for a child.

- Yeast overgrowth can cause thrush, a throat infection, or a skin infection that looks like diaper rash.
- The child may become allergic to the intestinal yeast *Candida albicans. Candida* allergy can cause a wide variety of symptoms, from congestion to eczema.[4]
- A constant allergic inflammation in the intestinal tract can create digestive disturbances such as gas and a general feeling of being bloated, and abdominal pain, constipation, or diarrhea.

- A yeast allergy may lead to other food allergies. Normally, the intestines keep out potential allergens such as food proteins, but a yeast-filled intestine becomes porous, allowing allergens to pass into the body. Allergies to yeasts and molds in food may develop, including the yeast in bread and crackers and the natural yeast on fruits, nuts, and seeds, on dried fruits such as raisins, and in commercial fruit juices. (The more "natural" a food is, the more likely it is to contain yeast. If you leave a bottle of apple cider without preservatives at room temperature for twenty-four hours, it will begin to ferment. Its natural yeast is multiplying and converting its sugar to alcohol and vinegar.) Vinegar, as a yeast by-product, can provoke an allergic reaction in a yeast-sensitive child, as can fermented soy sauce.

  Food yeasts don't grow in the body—they are not the same as *Candida,* the body yeast. But they can cause allergic reactions in yeast-sensitive children. Most cheeses, particularly the various blue cheeses, Stilton, and all hard cheeses, contain mold, and a yeast-sensitive child may react to them. Mold also grows quickly on strawberries and other fruits in the refrigerator, as well as on rotting foods in general. And molds are found everywhere outside—in dirt and dead leaves on the ground, for instance.

- *Candida albicans* can produce toxic substances.[5] C. Orian Truss, an Alabama physician, has speculated that these toxins may enter the bloodstream to create disturbances in other parts of the body. He has found that in certain people, a wide range of problems—including hormonal problems, emotional problems such as anxiety and depression, and neurological symptoms that may be mistakenly diagnosed as multiple sclerosis—clear up when the person's yeast infection is treated.[6] Truss's observations are controversial, but in my own practice I have had such good results with his treatment methods that I consider using them on all sick children who have been given several courses of antibiotics or who have become ill after one course (seven to ten days) of antibiotics.

For example, when I saw Fred, he had spent one-third of his young life taking antibiotics, but he had never been able to recover completely from a series of ear infections. His nose and chest were constantly congested.

Fred had been a healthy newborn and was fed breast milk and formula. At five months he started on solid foods, and at six months he had his first ear infection. He appeared to respond well to a course of antibiotics, but two months later his ear became infected again, and from then on his infection recurred every month. Drainage tubes in his ears slowed the rate of recurrence to every other month, but otherwise he made no improvement.

I confirmed my suspicion of *Candida* allergy by injecting a small dose of *Candida* extract into the skin of Fred's arm. This is a common technique for assessing immune response; people with normal immune responses will show a delayed reaction, developing a small red bump at the injection site in twenty-four to forty-eight hours. Fred, like other allergic people, developed an itchy red patch at the injection site in just ten minutes. Since his condition was serious, I recommended the following serious measures:

- A diet low in sugar and in foods containing yeast and molds. This wasn't easy for Fred or his parent. He couldn't eat bread, cheese, dried fruits, commercial fruit juices, or sweets of any kind. Because vinegar was also out, he couldn't eat mustard, mayonnaise, or catsup. Instead of bread, he ate rice crackers or matzoh. Because milk contains lactose, a sugar, he was limited to 1 cup a day. And because fruit contains sugar, he could have it only twice a day.
- We eliminated yeast-containing vitamins, and cut out all cereals containing malt. Malt is a product of the fermentation of grains with yeast and is a common flavoring in breakfast cereals. Fred could only eat unmalted cereals: oatmeal, puffed wheat, and puffed rice.
- Nystatin, a medication that kills yeast, and a freeze-dried mixture of lactobacillus bacteria to build up the levels of normal, yeast-controlling bacteria in his intestinal tract were prescribed.

Within two weeks, Fred's ear congestion was practically gone. But he hated his diet and was starting to think about how to cheat on it. Since he had made so much progress, we gradually liberalized his diet, restricting only sugar.

At the same time, we began giving him supplements of EFAs, zinc, and vitamins A and C. His hair and skin were somewhat dry, suggesting an EFA deficiency, so I recommended a tablespoon of flaxseed oil every day.

Fred's blood level of vitamin A was a bit low, and his hair zinc level was low as well. I recommended a yeast-free, hypoallergenic multivitamin and mineral supplement that would supply 10 milligrams of zinc and 5,000 units of vitamin A a day. The preparation, Basic Preventive, Jr., contained enough selenium, copper, iron, and manganese to offset the potential depleting effects of a zinc supplement on these minerals.

Because vitamin C has an antiallergic and, sometimes, even an immune system–stimulating effect, I recommended 1,000 milligrams of chewable vitamin C a day.

Over the next several months, Fred's ear infections gradually stopped and his congestion completely disappeared. He became more energetic and generally showed a great deal more vitality.

When your toddler has an ear infection, I recommend that you take the following steps:
- Don't push food on him. Let him eat at his own pace.
- Give him liquids frequently—follow the method described above for colds.
- Use Tylenol or aspirin for pain, not for fever.
- Use the prescribed antibiotic.
- Ask your pediatrician to prescribe Nystatin suspension—500,000 units to be taken three times a day as long as your child is on the antibiotic and for one week after.
- Give your child *Lactobacillus acidophilus* and *Lactobacillus bifidus*, both of which combat yeast.

I recommend a half teaspoon of each twice a day while your child is infected and for one to two weeks after any course of antibiotics. (It is best to give these to your child as supplements, as commercial yogurt may not be an adequate source of *Lactobacillus*—by the time you buy it, most of the active yogurt culture may have died. As a test, try using a spoonful of commercial yogurt as a starter to make homemade yogurt; if it doesn't work, the bacteria are dead.)

Acidophilus milk does supply some active bacteria, but I prefer powdered, freeze-dried *Lactobacillus:* Primedophilus and Primeplex from Klaire Laboratories, and Ultradophilus and Bifido Factor from Natren have all worked well for my patients. Be careful about what you buy; some commercial *Lactobacillus* products are worthless—they contain almost no viable organisms.

You can mix freeze-dried *acidophilus* and *bifidus* into milk, yogurt, or other food. Primedophilus, with a sweetish taste, is perhaps the most palatable. These preparations are particularly effective against antibiotic-induced diarrhea.

Two other yeast-controlling preparations, garlic oil and caprylic acid, aren't really suitable for toddlers. Garlic oil is quite strong in taste and smell (the deodorized product doesn't work) and you need to take a lot of it. Caprylic acid, a derivative of coconut oil, is widely available, but it can be irritating and should be taken only in pill form. Toddlers generally aren't ready to swallow pills.

- Continue giving him his usual doses of flaxseed oil and vitamin C.

RESPIRATORY-TRACT INFECTIONS

I've found the following approach generally effective for *recurrent* or *chronic* respiratory-tract infections.

- Absolutely follow my basic meal plan for optimal nutrition.
- Your child probably has one or more nutritional deficiencies; most common are omega-3 EFA, vitamins A, C, or B-6, zinc, and/or iron deficiency. Give him the following:

EFAs: flaxseed oil	1 Tb daily
Vitamin A: cod-liver oil	1 tsp daily
Vitamin C: chewable	
Ages 1–3	500 mg a day
Ages 3–5	1,000 mg a day
Vitamin B-6:	25 mg a day in a chewable B complex
Zinc: oyster-rich seafood stew	Twice a week
Iron: calf's liver	Once or twice a week

- Search for allergies by following the directions in Chapter 4, page 86. If a child has had lots of antibiotics, an allergy to the body yeast *Candida albicans* is likely. If your child hasn't had any antibiotics, he is most likely to be allergic to milk, wheat, or house dust.

A serious yeast problem usually requires treatment by a physician who knows how to treat it effectively.

In addition, you can follow the suggestions in the previous section, Ear Infections, on how to provide your toddler with a diet free of sugar, yeast, and mold. And give your toddler half a teaspoon each of *Lactobacillus acidophilus* and *Lactobacillus bifidus* (see above, under Ear Infections) twice a day during the infection and for two weeks after any course of antibiotics.

ALLERGIES

ASTHMA AND ECZEMA

These allergic problems can devastate a toddler. Their symptoms can also be misleading. Some children with chronic coughs may actually have asthma, even though they don't wheeze or have a problem with shortness of breath. Your first step in treatment is to follow the instructions in Chapter 4, page 86, for evaluating your child's diet for food allergies, paying special attention to foods containing milk, yeast, and molds. (See p. 126 under Ear Infections above for a description of foods containing yeast and molds.)

In allergies, as in recurrent infections, deficiencies in certain nutrients contribute to a malfunction of the immune system. One of the main problems is likely to be *EFAs,* which are crucial to the production of the prostaglandins that regulate all immune functioning. For omega-3s, give your toddler 1 tablespoon of flaxseed oil a day. You can start this right away and continue it as you go through your allergy-detection work.

Your child is likely to have a problem with omega-6 EFAs that involves more than just a dietary deficiency. In fact, back in 1931 Arild Hansen, a Minnesota pediatrician, found that children with eczema had abnormal levels of some omega-6 EFAs in their blood. His work attracted some attention until cortisone became available for treatment, at which point it was ignored. But cortisone can produce terrible side effects, such as diabetes, high blood pressure, brittle bones, and atrophy of the skin. In 1981 two British dermatologists replicated Hansen's results and found that evening primrose oil was effective in relieving a group of severely afflicted patients.[7]

Evening primrose and black currant oils, as we have seen, contain GLA, an EFA that is created in the body as an intermediate step in the production of prostaglandins. Every step of the prostaglandin production process is controlled by enzymes. A key enzyme in converting the main omega-6 EFA, linoleic acid (LA), into GLA is D-6-D; I call it the *Delta Force.* In children and adults with allergic eczema, asthma, and hay fever, the Delta Force appears to be much less active than normal. As a result, prostaglandin production is short-circuited.

Primrose oil is sold in 500-milligram capsules; I recommend Efamol brand, part of Murdoch Pharmaceuticals' Nature's Way line. (Beware of products masquerading as primrose oil; they contain little or no GLA. Stick with Efamol brand.) If primrose oil is unavailable, you may use black currant oil, also a good source of GLA. Although both oils are expensive, you need only use a small amount.

Start your toddler on two capsules of primrose oil a day; since he probably isn't ready to swallow them, the best thing is to cut them open and rub the oil on his skin. It will be absorbed through his skin into his body. Black currant oil capsules contain as much or more GLA as primrose oil; you can rub one of these into your toddler's skin each day. If he doesn't improve, add a capsule, up to four a day.

A less effective, but also less expensive, alternative to evening primrose oil or black currant oil is to provide a lot of LA so that at least some of it will be converted to GLA. If you choose this method, give your child 1 to 3 tablespoons of safflower or sunflower oil a day.

A child with omega-6 conversion problems may also have a deficiency in the co-factor vitamins and minerals that are essential in helping the Delta Force do its work of converting LA to prostaglandins. Vitamin A, certain B vitamins, magnesium, zinc, and iron are particularly important. (Food sources of the co-factor minerals were listed in Chapter 4.) Unfortunately, though, food allergies may make it difficult for your child to get enough of these vitamins and minerals in his diet. The answer to this problem, of course, is supplements:

Vitamin A: cod-liver oil	1 tsp daily
Vitamins B-2, -3, and -6: a hypoallergenic B-complex, free of sugar, starch, yeast, and artificial coloring	Should supply 25 mg of vitamin B-6 daily
Zinc: zinc lozenge	10 mg of zinc daily
Iron: ferrous sulfate liquid	15 mg of iron daily
Magnesium	6 mg per pound of weight daily: 240 mg for a 40-lb child
Magnesium citrate liquid	About 1 Tb daily
Milk of magnesia	About 1½ tsp daily

Magnesium is hard to find in a form suitable for young children. Magnesium citrate, a widely used laxative, seems to be absorbed best; to prevent a laxative effect, I have recommended a sublaxative dose. Milk of magnesia, containing magnesium hydroxide, is second-best.

In addition to being a co-factor mineral, magnesium is an antihistamine. Histamine is a natural chemical that when released into the blood as part of an allergic reaction causes many of the symptoms of allergy. Animal studies have shown that magnesium deficiency increases the amount of histamine released into the blood. Magnesium has not been extensively studied in relation to childhood asthma or eczema, but some adults with magnesium deficiency show high levels of histamine that decrease when they take magnesium. And young adults with asthma have lower levels of magnesium in their blood than their nonasthmatic peers. The most common drugs used in controlling allergy symptoms are the antihistamines—magnesium may work nearly as well.

Vitamin C in high doses is also an effective antihistamine. The doses that can produce this effect, 500 to 5,000 milligrams a day, are quite safe, even for toddlers, and vitamin C comes in chewable tablets. The main side effect of an excess of either magnesium or vitamin C is diarrhea, which will stop when the dosage is reduced.

Maria is a good example of the successful nutritional treatment of eczema. When I first saw her, she was a sad 3½-year-old. Her parents both had allergies—her mother, asthma; her father, hay fever. As a baby, Maria was fed a milk-based formula. Her eczema started at 3 months. It improved when she was switched to a soy-based formula, but the minute she began eating solid foods it returned.

Maria's doctor prescribed a cortisone cream to control her eczema, but when I saw her she still had red, itchy, scaling patches on her chest, arms, and legs. And even where there was no eczema her skin was dry.

I recommended that her parents rub two capsules a day of evening primrose oil directly on her eczema. This reduced the symptoms enough so that the cortisone cream was applied three times a week instead of three times a day.

Since Maria's skin was still dry, I decided that she probably needed extra omega-3 EFAs as well. (The Delta Force is also crucial to the conversion of the key omega-3 EFA, LNA, to prostaglandins. In fact, Hansen successfully used flaxseed oil to treat eczema in his child patients.) I had her parents give her 1 tablespoon a day of flaxseed oil in juice, plus 1 teaspoon of mint-flavored cod-liver oil. Over the next several weeks her skin and hair became more lustrous and her eczema continued to improve.

I also recommended supplements of some co-factor minerals and vitamins: a zinc lozenge supplying 10 milligrams a day, magnesium citrate supplying 200 milligrams a day, a chewable multivitamin supplying B vitamins, and a chewable vitamin C supplying 500 milligrams a day. The magnesium and C worked as antihistamines as well as co-factors.

Because Maria was on a milk-free diet, I had her parents give her 600 milligrams of chewable calcium carbonate a day with her meals.

For other children with eczema, I've had to advise elimination diets, allergy desensitization, and treatment for *Candida albicans* problems. Maria was lucky; she responded to EFA and co-factor nutrients, plus calcium.

BEHAVIORAL PROBLEMS

Toddlers can develop all the behavioral problems common in school-age children: They can be hyperactive, prone to temper tantrums, and moody. (As we saw in Chapter 4, these behaviors can become evident while a child is still an infant.) While such behavior may not be as big a problem at this stage as it will be in school, it's a good idea to identify and treat the symptoms now. In my practice, I have treated many difficult children, and I've found that with nutritional treatment, the personalities of difficult preschoolers often change amazingly for the better. Once a child is over seven years old, though, and patterns of aggressive, manipulative, or self-destructive behavior are well established, nutritional treatment may no longer be enough.

A child who is difficult and behaves badly creates an unhappy situation for himself. His attitudes and actions produce negative feedback that, in turn, can make his behavior worse. He develops a poor self-image that is likely to be reinforced in school by teachers who find him hard to handle. In his excellent book *The Difficult Child*, Dr. Stanley Turecki describes the difficult child as very active, easily distracted, poor at adapting to new situations, irregular in his patterns of sleeping and eating, moody, and very sensitive to such external stimuli as noise, smells, and bright lights. Turecki points out that some children show only some of these traits, while others are figuratively "parent killers."

Hyperactivity and *attention-deficit disorder* are the most common labels applied to these children's symptoms, but as diagnoses they are really spurious. Hyperactivity is not a disease; it is merely a description of the behavior of some types of difficult children. In the pages that follow, I may use the terms *hyperactive* and *difficult* interchangeably when referring to children with all or some of Turecki's traits. Turecki outlines a behavioral program for treating such children, but at the toddler age a nutritional program may be even more effective. Irritable, distractible, hypersensitive toddlers are not just poorly buffered psychologically; they are also poorly buffered biochemically. That means that they respond excessively to minor changes in their body's physiological state. They are often hypersensitive to foods and to nutritional supplements. Sometimes they are truly allergic, but often their hypersensitivities are biochemical.

Difficult children tend to eat more sugar than other children, and their parents often notice that the youngsters' behavior deteriorates after they've eaten sweets. Whether sugar alone causes this is a matter of controversy, though. In tests at the National Institutes of Health, sugar-sensitive children who were

given sugared water didn't become hyperactive or irritable, suggesting that some other factor must be at work.

A genetic factor is undoubtedly involved. Difficult children
often have a parent who was or is hyperactive, restless, or extremely moody. A family history of alcoholism is more common
among children diagnosed as hyperactive than among other children.

Dr. Ben Feingold, a California pediatrician, found that some
hyperactive children are biochemically hypersensitive to salicylates, aspirinlike substances in foods, and food dyes. This is not
a true allergy; rather, the nervous system is sensitive to exposure
to salicylates. A National Institutes of Health panel concluded
that only a small fraction of hyperactive children were hypersensitive to salicylates but thought the frequency of salicylate sensitivity was great enough to warrant a trial of a low-salicylate diet in
selected cases.[8] Recent data suggest that the Feingold diet may
not be restrictive enough and that continued salicylate consumption despite the diet may impair its effectiveness.

Almonds and other nuts, as well as apples and citrus fruits
contain natural salicylates. Salicylates are especially concentrated in dried fruits. Many food additives, particularly artificial
food coloring and such preservatives as BHT, are salicylates. My
experience is that artificial salicylates (food dyes and preservatives) tend to cause more problems than do natural salicylates and
that the consumption of sugar with salicylates causes a more
intense response; this has been noted by others as well.[9] I have
found the following measures helpful with difficult, temperamental, hyperactive, impulsive toddlers.

- Keep sugar, candy, ice cream, cake, and other high-sugar foods
  out of your child's diet altogether. Don't keep any in the house
  and ask relatives and friends not to offer them. Also limit foods
  high in natural sugar: don't serve him any dried fruits. Limit
  him to 4 ounces of fruit juice and two pieces of fresh fruit a day.
  Don't serve artificially colored, flavored, or preserved food.
- Follow the diet plan in Chapter 5 and the recipes in Chapter 10.
  But keep in mind that children with behavioral problems often
  have very irregular rhythms. They may not eat three meals a
  day, and they may awaken earlier and go to sleep later than
  other children. Give your child frequent snacks of high-protein

foods such as carrot sticks with nut butter, or crackers with nut butter or cheese.

- *EFA supplements* may have a calming effect. If you are following the toddler diet plan outlined in Chapter 5, you are already giving your child 1 tablespoon of flaxseed oil (or substitute 1 teaspoon of cod-liver oil or 2 tablespoons of walnut oil) a day to supply omega-3 EFAs. If you haven't started, start now, and pay attention to your child's behavior, his sleep patterns, and the dryness of his skin. Notice how thirsty he is. Children who are restless, have dry skin, and are excessively thirsty are likely to benefit from the right EFA supplement, and you should notice some positive change within two weeks of starting flaxseed oil or its substitutes.

But difficult children can be biochemically unpredictable, with strange or even negative responses to nutritional supplements. If your difficult child's skin seems to become dryer with flaxseed oil or its substitutes, or if he becomes thirstier, stop the flaxseed oil and substitute 1 tablespoon of safflower oil. Or rub two capsules (1 gram) of primrose oil or two capsules of black currant oil into his skin each day. Or, keep giving him flaxseed oil or cod-liver or walnut oil in its place and rub two to three capsules of primrose or black currant oil into his skin daily. If he becomes thirstier after starting this program, or if his skin becomes dryer or his behavior deteriorates in any way, discontinue it. In my experience, about 80 percent of hyperactive children benefit from EFAs, with equal numbers responding to flaxseed oil and to primrose or black currant oil.

Georgia, for instance, drove her parents crazy. She could act like an angel, then, for no good reason, throw a terrible temper tantrum. When I examined her, I found small rough patches on her cheeks where the skin was covered with tiny bumps. On the soles of her feet, her skin peeled. All these symptoms stopped when I put her on the toddler diet with flaxseed oil.

Deborah was harder to deal with. She was a wild child, with violent mood swings—a toddler Jekyll and Hyde. She turned her bed upside down every night, had a voracious appetite, and was constantly thirsty. The toddler diet with flaxseed oil seemed to have no effect on these symptoms. I suggested that her mother rub three capsules a day of primrose oil into her skin. Within forty-eight hours Deborah's thirst had diminished; within a week, her appetite and sleep patterns had become more normal. She remained wild, but with love and patience (fatty acids can't do everything) she became more stable as she grew into school age.

- Difficult children need more magnesium and calcium than other children. Possibly, they excrete more magnesium because of their constantly high adrenaline levels. Whatever the mechanism, their magnesium deficit in turn lowers their blood calcium levels. The two deficits lead to twitchiness, insomnia, and abdominal pain.

  Snacks of nuts and nut butters are a good way to provide magnesium and stabilize blood sugar. Don't give your child too much milk or cottage cheese to supply calcium; an excess of calcium and vitamin D will actually increase the amount of magnesium he needs. Limit dairy products to 16 ounces a day.

  You can try one of the magnesium supplements described on page 132, 6 milligrams per pound of his body weight every day. If he drinks very little milk, add about 500 milligrams of calcium a day. If he has a problem with sleep, try giving him the magnesium at bedtime; it should have a calming effect.

- *B-vitamins* are tricky for this group. Although scientists don't yet know why, vitamin B supplements, including ordinary multivitamins, can actually increase a child's behavior problems. If your child is taking a multivitamin, stop it for two weeks to see whether he becomes less jittery and aggressive or sleeps better. Sometimes individual B-vitamins, usually B-6 or B-1, are helpful. Try 10 milligrams a day of vitamin B-6 or vitamin B-1 alone, then add a B complex.

- *Lead*, in higher than average levels in the blood, can be associated with hyperactivity. This is most often found in poorer inner-city neighborhoods, but recently high lead levels have also been found in middle-class children living in older homes or apartment buildings with pipes whose joints are soldered with lead.[10] It has been recommended that cold-water taps be run for three minutes or more each morning to clear the pipes of lead leached in overnight, and that water from the hot-water tap never be drunk or used in cooking. Iron or zinc deficiency

or a diet low in calcium increases a child's susceptibility to lead
poisoning.

• *Allergies* contribute to a wide variety of behavioral disturbances in children—about 70 percent of hyperactive children
are allergic to some kinds of food and inhalants (the pollen,
dust, and mold that are inhaled along with air when we
breathe). Allergies may just make the child uncomfortable and
irritable, but in some cases they seem to directly affect the
brain, possibly producing localized swelling or chemicals that
affect brain function.

Controlled studies have shown that food allergies play a significant role in hyperactivity.[11] In a Texas study twelve severely
hyperactive children who had not responded to any therapy were
tested with a sophisticated procedure called the Brain Stem
Evoked Potential (BSEP). They all had abnormal electrical activity in their brains. After trials were conducted to discover the
foods to which they were allergic and they stopped eating them,
their BSEPs became normal and their behavior improved.[12]

I would recommend a food trial to find out what food or foods
your child is allergic to. Usually a child is allergic to several
different foods, but the most common single culprit is milk. Sometimes, the "allergy" turns out to be a hypersensitivity to salicylates, as Dr. Feingold described.

If a hyperactive child has been given a lot of antibiotics, he
almost always has a problem with yeast. Antiyeast treatment has
resulted in dramatic improvements in children whose behavior has
deteriorated after a course of antibiotics.

For instance, Bobby and his twin brother were healthy at birth
after a normal, full-term pregnancy. But they were hard to handle, and they both seemed to have allergies. Their main symptom was chronic nasal congestion, but Bobby also developed a
series of ear infections that were treated with several different
antibiotics.

As the two boys entered the "terrible twos," they drove their
mother, a registered nurse, to distraction. Her pediatrician felt
the boys' problems were simply expressions of their personalities.

When the twins turned three, Bobby's behavior deteriorated,
while his brother's improved. Bobby was aggressive and moody;
he bit, kicked, and cried easily. He was a restless sleeper and a

poor eater and was very easily frustrated. He was also impulsive and easily distracted. In short, he became a holy terror. His pediatrician suggested the drug Ritalin, frequently prescribed for hyperactive children, but recommended waiting until Bobby was in school.

Bobby's mother suggested taking him to the Gesell Institute for an evaluation. Her pediatrician scoffed, but she did bring the child in and I saw him. His antibiotic history was so strong, and was so clearly the difference between Bobby and his twin, that I recommended six months of a yeast-free diet and a two-month course of Nystatin treatment. Bobby's mother had already eliminated sugar from his diet. Now she cut out cheese, yeast breads and crackers, vitamins made from yeast, unpeeled fresh fruit, dried fruit, and commercial fruit juices. She prepared her own yeast-free bread and fresh orange juice.

After six weeks, Bobby was like a new child. Everyone—his parents, his relatives, even his pediatrician—recognized the changes in his personality. (For more on yeasts, and a yeast-free diet, see Chapter 7.)

Andy, though, was a little boy with a more serious problem— in fact, he may never completely recover. At two, Andy was diagnosed as *autistic*, meaning that he did not communicate with the outside world. Some children appear to be autistic almost from birth. Others, like Andy, start out looking normal. By two, Andy had begun to speak. Then he had a series of respiratory infections, for which he was given antibiotics. Within a few weeks after his second ear infection, he stopped talking. He became much less responsive, and would grow violent if he were thwarted in any way. His appetite became voracious. His parents took him to a series of specialists, one of whom eventually diagnosed him as autistic.

Andy's parents chose a program of calculated permissiveness: They wouldn't force him to do anything. Instead, they would try to shape his world to conform to him. They brought in mother's helpers and volunteers to cater to him.

Slowly, Andy became less difficult and more predictable. But when, at three, he was given another round of antibiotics for an ear infection, he completely regressed and lost all self-control. He had seizurelike falling spells and developed chronic diarrhea.

A friend of Andy's mother who was being treated for a yeast-allergy problem suggested that Andy might have a similar allergy. His mother took him to a clinical ecologist, a doctor specializing in allergies and other hypersensitive reactions to the environment. This doctor skin-tested Andy and told his mother that he had multiple food allergies. He suggested that she stop giving Andy any food and substitute Vivonex, a hypoallergenic but sugar-containing food substitute. At first, Andy's behavior improved; he seemed less "spacey." But then he regressed again. At that point, his mother brought him to me.

My assessment was that antibiotics were the main cause of Andy's problems. By killing off the good bacteria in his intestines, the antibiotics had allowed an overgrowth of yeast that had damaged the intestinal lining, creating multiple food allergies. I also thought that the yeast overgrowth might have had a toxic effect on Andy's body, leading to biochemical disturbances that could account for some of his behavior.

I had Andy stop Vivonex and start eating seafood and vegetables. We experimented with several diets and found that he did best on rice, vegetables, tofu, and some fish. We also tried various drugs to decrease the yeast in his intestines. Andy reacted poorly to most of them, but he was able to tolerate Capricin. This over-the-counter coconut-oil derivative tastes awful when removed from its capsule. Fortunately, unlike 99 percent of toddlers, Andy could swallow anything that was shoved down his throat! We added two *Lactobacillus* preparations: an *acidophilus* and a *bifidus*.

Andy also had an extensive metabolic evaluation that uncovered a problem in digestion—undigested fat and starch were present in his stool. He had deficiencies of vitamins A and B-6, and magnesium, copper, zinc, iron, and selenium. He couldn't tolerate a B-vitamin supplement; it made him more aggressive and interfered with his sleep. But he did well with supplements of magnesium, cod-liver oil, flaxseed oil, primrose oil, zinc, copper, selenium, and iron. When he stopped these, he withdrew and began falling apart again.

When I first saw Andy, his face had a dull expression, his tongue lolled out of his mouth, and he had dark puffy rings around his eyes. He couldn't walk by himself. After a year of intense treatment, he had become affectionate and expressive and could walk and run. From a distance, he looked quite normal, although he still didn't talk. Best of all, though, a repeat psychological assessment indicated that *Andy isn't autistic*. His ability to learn is excellent, and he has now begun to speak.

Few children have problems as extreme as Andy's, but his story underlines the importance of the points I've been stressing in this chapter.

- *Antibiotics can have a devastating effect on some children.*
- *A yeast infection can create severe allergic and, possibly, biochemical disturbances.* Those of you who want to know more about this should read *The Missing Diagnosis* by C. Orian Truss, M.D., and *The Yeast Connection* by William Crook, M.D.

   I feel strongly that all children who take antibiotics should be given treatment to normalize their intestinal flora. This includes a low-sugar, high-fiber diet and both *Lactobacillus acidophilus* and *Lactobacillus bifidus* preparations. If the child is given antibiotics again, or if he's allergic to start with, I would give him Nystatin to inhibit yeast growth.

Finally, the stories of Andy and the other children I've told in this chapter also underline my experience that even the most severe behavioral disturbances in children may respond to nutritional treatment.

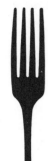

Ages Five to Twelve:
Feeding Your School-Age Child
for Extra Immunity

7

The school-age child is moving out beyond her home, and this means new experiences. At school, your child will encounter a new, more disciplined environment that even a day-care center may not have prepared her for. New stresses will become part of her life—she'll face pressures to learn, to compete, and to conform to unfamiliar rules. Stress will test her immune system, and so will the barrage of new viruses and bacteria she will encounter, especially if she hasn't spent time in a nursery school or day-care center. But the foods you feed her, and the eating habits you reinforce, can keep her a vibrantly healthy child whose body is well able to cope with new challenges.

Eating habits are especially important at this age because for the first time she will have to cope on her own with other people's eating patterns and that modern menace, junk food. In her preschool years, it was relatively easy to control her access to junk food, although she was certainly exposed to it on TV and on outings with other parents. Now, she's on her own much more. She will eat and sleep at friends' houses, and discover that other kids eat candy and ice cream, Twinkies and Oreos—not to mention potato chips—at home. She may also find that at meals they eat fried foods, or a lot of meat. Perhaps for the first time, she will question your menus.

How do you cope?

By following the sensible basic nutrition plan in this chapter, you'll keep your child's diet high in essential fatty acids (EFAs) and in the co-factor nutrients that will help her body metabolize EFAs: vitamins A, B-6, C, E and the minerals magnesium, zinc, copper, and selenium. EFA metabolism, you may recall from Chapter 1, produces the prostaglandins that keep her immune system, as well as her cardiorespiratory and nervous systems, working well.

She'll also have plenty of iron and a good supply of the antioxidants that protect her immune system as it does its work: vitamins A, C, E, B-2, and B-3, and zinc, copper, manganese, and sulfur. Antioxidants protect against the effects of radiation, help the body defend itself against the toxins in other environmental pollutants, and provide important protection against free radicals, which are found in heat-damaged oils used in fast-food outlets. Free radicals damage cells, including immune cells, and they turn up in French fries, hamburgers, deep-fried fish, or chicken nuggets—in short, in all deep-fried food, whether prepared by somebody's mother or at McDonald's.

If necessary, in addition to the flaxseed oil or walnut or cod-liver oil you'll give her every day to provide her with omega-3 EFAs, she can take supplements of vitamins C and E to provide an extra boost of antioxidants, or she can take magnesium to correct a deficiency that could contribute to allergies.

Away from home she's going to be exposed to all kinds of anti-nutrients—the sugar, fats, salt, and phosphates that interfere with prostaglandin production and so undermine her immune system. Soft drinks and commercial pastries are loaded with sugar, but sugar also turns up in peanut butter, catsup, and other spreads and condiments, and in such lunch meats as turkey roll. Fats—especially hydrogenated or partially hydrogenated oils— are added to commercial baked goods, sauces, lunch meats, and virtually all manufactured snacks and foods. Hydrogenation destroys the essential fatty acids in otherwise healthy oils. Fats and sugar, which provide neither vitamins nor minerals, are major causes of obesity. And they may increase the body's need for certain nutrients to help it undo the damage they do.

Manufactured foods are also usually very high in salt. Check the label on a can of soup—it may contain almost 1,000 milligrams of sodium, as much as your child should consume in the entire day. Canned or bottled spaghetti sauces—almost any food in a can or bottle, for that matter—many breakfast cereals, most snack foods, lunch meats and cheeses, and many baked goods have salt added. Yet children already get all the salt they need from foods in which it occurs naturally. Added salt only contributes to high blood pressure, while depleting the body's supplies of magnesium by triggering its excretion into the urine.

When your child drinks most soft drinks, she'll consume phosphates, chemicals added to balance the carbonation. Phosphates are also widely used as preservatives in manufactured food. Wherever they're used, they block her body's ability to absorb calcium and magnesium from the nutritious food she eats at home.

But take heart: you can still control *most* of the food she eats, including her school lunches. If her basic diet is sound, a little junk food once in a while won't hurt. And, if she's used to a low-fat, low-sugar diet, she's not likely to crave high-sugar sweets or deep-fried chicken nuggets. She may very well find them too sweet, too greasy. When the kids go to Burger King, she might even fix a salad at the salad bar and just nibble on a few fries. I'll help you develop a strategy to use on the days when she comes home from a friend's house and says, "Sally's mom lets her have Devil Dogs and Pepsi every afternoon!"

WHAT TO FEED YOUR SCHOOL-AGE CHILD

Nutritional needs don't change much at this age. To ensure normal growth, a healthy immune system, and optimum intellectual development, she will still need a balanced, varied diet of foods low in sugar and fat and high in vitamins, minerals, and essential fatty acids. She should have three meals and a snack every day.
- a high-protein breakfast
- a brown-bag lunch you prepare at home
- an after-school snack
- a family supper

BREAKFAST

Never skip breakfast. Your child should get at least one-third of the nutrients she needs every day from this meal, and it should be high in protein, not carbohydrates. Protein lowers the levels of a brain chemical called serotonin, which plays a role in making people sleepy. Most children respond to a high-protein breakfast by remaining alert all morning long. A high-carbohydrate breakfast, on the other hand, makes them (and you) drowsy because it enhances the brain's synthesis of serotonin. It's worth getting up fifteen minutes earlier so that you'll have enough time to fix a good breakfast.

Protein

Eggs are a good source of protein, but serve them boiled or poached; don't fry or scramble them. Frying and scrambling oxidizes the cholesterol in the egg yolk, producing chemicals that damage blood vessels. Boiled or poached eggs are delicious on whole wheat toast.

Tofu has no cholesterol, so you can stir-fry it or scramble it. It's a good breakfast food, and this is a good time to introduce your child to it. (See Chapter 10.)

Homemade cereal provides protein and many vitamins and minerals; homemade oatmeal, granola, and Swiss muesli are all delicious. (See Chapter 10.) *Seeds and nuts* help raise the protein and mineral content of cereals; you'll use them in granola and muesli, but you can also mix them into oatmeal or any sugar-free commercial cereal. (Check the toddler breakfast menus in Chapter 5 for tips on these and other breakfast choices such as Sesame Waffles, that your child will still enjoy. Also, check the information on pp. 110–11 on convenience foods.)

Leftovers can be good sources of protein, although most Americans don't like fish or beans for breakfast.

Milk provides protein and calcium. (*Note:* Your child doesn't need to drink whole milk any longer. It's time to serve her low-fat milk and yogurt, if she'll take them.)

Definitely avoid bacon! This traditional breakfast staple has too much fat, salt, and cancer-causing nitrates. Ditto ham and sausage.

Vitamin C

Fresh fruit and orange or grapefruit juice are important sources of vitamin C and should be part of every breakfast. Fresh fruit makes cereals deliciously sweet.

Carbohydrates

Carbohydrates should not be the main part of breakfast because, as I said above, they create drowsiness rather than alertness. But as an adjunct to high-protein foods, 100 percent whole wheat bread or toast is delicious. Check the label to make sure *whole* wheat flour is the first ingredient listed (stone-ground whole wheat flour is best). *Wheat flour* is just a euphemism for refined white flour; *unbleached flour* is highly refined. Avoid them. The wheat can also be sprouted or cracked. Other whole grains, such as rye, barley, and corn, make excellent ingredients. A crunchy, multigrain bread makes terrific toast.

Serve toast either under an egg, or with stir-fried or scrambled tofu, or with nut butter, sugar-free apple butter, or sugar-free fruit conserve. Don't use butter or margarine—the first is pure fat, the second pure hydrogenated fat. Naturally, you won't serve commercial sweet rolls, muffins, coffee cake, or Danish.

At eight, Justin was eating a soft roll and glass of orange juice for breakfast. By lunchtime he was famished and ate everything on the school lunch menu, including dessert. He wasn't doing well in school; he seemed spaced-out and sleepy and didn't read well. Since he perked up for recess, his teacher thought he was just not motivated to learn. At night, though, it was a different story— Justin was rambunctious and lively. He had a hard time falling asleep.

It was obvious to me that Justin's body rhythms were out of sync with his world. My solution was to put him on a high-protein breakfast of eggs, tofu, meat, milk, yogurt, or cottage cheese. Most carbohydrates—pasta, whole-grain bread, vegetables, and fruits—were shifted to supper, when he ate no meat.

I also had Justin's parents cut out TV at night and begin to structure the time in ways that would help him settle down to a good night's sleep. In addition to a family meal, Justin's homework, and a warm bath, they began giving him ten minutes or more of undivided attention every night.

Within two weeks, Justin became more alert in school. His reading—and his grades—improved. And he slept better at night.

Sharing time with your children is an important way of expressing love, that all-important "invisible nutrient" children need. There is no age limit on the need for people who love each other to spend time together—your child will need this special time-sharing until he's at least eighteen—and perhaps older.

Is there always enough time to give your child some undivided attention? Yes. If you think about how to spend the time that's available, rather than worry about how little time you have, you'll find there is time even if you have several children. One family of three boys gave each boy ten or twenty minutes of "exclusive private time" every day. Each boy could call his shot: sharing supper preparations, playing, reading, a brisk walk, or a quiet conversation. *Time* is the most precious gift we can give to those we love.

Fiber

At this age fiber becomes important because your child can get it only from her food, and breakfast is a good meal at which to provide it. (Youngsters under five can't tolerate fiber well, so I haven't recommended it before.) Fiber feeds the good bacteria in the intestine that keep yeast from getting out of hand (see p. 89 for a thorough discussion of what yeast can do when it gets out of hand). Fiber also helps prevent bowel cancer and also appears to help prevent heart disease later in life.

What is fiber? Simply stated, it's the part of plants that isn't digested by enzymes in the stomach and intestines. It comes in two varieties, *soluble* and *insoluble.* Insoluble fiber doesn't even dissolve in powerful stomach acid. It is coarse and has the effect of scrubbing the intestine, helping to prevent bowel cancer. Wheat bran is full of insoluble fiber.

Soluble fiber does dissolve in digestive juices to form a soft gel. Your child doesn't digest it but the good bacteria in her intestine do; it supports their growth. This bacterial digestion of soluble fiber releases substances that can lower cholesterol, kill harmful bacteria and yeasts, and nourish the large intestine.

Fruits, beans, and oat bran all contain soluble fiber—oat bran is the best source. The typical American diet doesn't supply enough fiber, so it's vital that you serve fiber-rich foods. Just make sure that you give your child a lot of water to drink whenever you serve her a high-fiber food. Without water to dilute it, fiber can actually be constipating. Children who have frequent or chronic abdominal pain, with or without accompanying constipation, often benefit from a high-fiber diet.

When Sally's pediatrician sent her to me at age eight, she complained every day of stomachaches. She moved her bowels every other day, and her stools were hard.

Since the pediatrician could find no organic cause for Sally's abdominal pains, he chalked them up to anxiety and stress. Sally's diet was better than most, but far from perfect: she ate a lot of chicken and fish, salads, eggs, yogurt, cheese, and bananas and fruit juices. Although low in sugar and high in nutrients, this diet provided few foods rich in fiber.

I asked her mother to substitute fresh fruits, such as apples and berries, for fruit juice, and add whole grains to her diet, substituting brown rice and whole wheat bread for white rice and bread. She ate more beans, especially in salads. (Most basic salad ingredients—lettuce, cucumbers, and celery—are 99 percent water and, therefore, very low in fiber.) She also ate beans as a protein substitute for meat. For breakfast, she began eating oatmeal with added oat bran and fresh fruit.

Within three weeks, Sally's abdominal pains had stopped and she was having normal daily bowel movements.

I could have treated Sally with psyllium husks (the basis for Metamucil, used for "regularity" by many older adults) to provide fiber, but whenever possible it's better to change a child's eating habits to prevent her problem from recurring rather than simply to dose her with supplements.

The most important supplement is flaxseed oil; breakfast is the ideal time to give your child the 1 tablespoon of flaxseed oil that most children continue to need each day. Mix it into her cereal or juice, or give it to her straight. (Keep this oil in the refrigerator after you've opened it.) You may substitute 1 teaspoon of cod-liver oil or 2 tablespoons of walnut oil if flaxseed oil is unavailable.

LUNCH

Can you trust the lunch served at your child's school? Unless she goes to a special school indeed, the odds are you can't. Even when schools try to serve "balanced meals" that include vegetables, they generally contain too much sugar, fat, and salt, and too little in the way of such key minerals as zinc and copper. Besides, hot lunches sit in steam tables while the heat destroys vitamins by the minute. (The food is therefore more nutritious in the first lunch period than the second or third.)

You're better off making your child's lunch yourself. Sandwiches are delicious, convenient, and supply a good mixture of ingredients. Whole wheat pita (pocket) bread not only stands up under all kinds of fillings, but it is made without sugar or oil. Whole wheat bread, in addition to being 100 percent whole wheat (see above under Breakfast), should be made without preservatives and hydrogenated or partially hydrogenated oils. This eliminates all the major brands of commercial bread. Try baking your own bread or buying it in a good bakery or health-food store. Since shortening helps make and keep bread moist, it is virtually always used—try to find bread made with unhydrogenated safflower or soy oil. Some brands to look for: Bread for Life, Food for Life, Shiloh Farms (health-food stores), Stroehmann's Grain Bin (supermarkets). Keep it fresh in the refrigerator or freezer; to restore its natural flavor, toast it lightly.

Spreads and Fillers

You can fill whole wheat bread or pita pockets with plain, home-cooked meat, fish, or poultry; nut or apple butter; falafel and hummus with alfalfa sprouts and grated cheese; or with salmon, tuna, or chicken salad with chopped celery. Keep away from commercial lunch meats—bologna, salami, turkey roll, pressed ham, and so forth are chock-full of fat, sugar, and salt.

Spreads. Don't use commercial spreads such as catsup or mayonnaise. In fact, no matter how many times your school-age child tells you that his friends' mothers let them use catsup, keep it out of your kitchen altogether. It is full of sugar. (There is one exception, described in Chapter 10.)

Commercial mayonnaise is a dangerous food because it is usually made with partially hydrogenated vegetable oils and egg yolks (the partially hydrogenated oils are more nutritionally harmful than the 10 milligrams or so of cholesterol in the egg yolks). But you can get tofu-based mayonnaise in health-food stores. It's the best commercial mayonnaise because it supplies protein and minerals and is free of destructive fats. Nasoya is a good brand. In some locations, you can also find egg-yolk mayonnaise made with pure, unhydrogenated soy oil (Cain's brand).

The best mayonnaise, though, is homemade—see Chapter 10 for both tofu and egg-yolk versions. Homemade flaxseed-oil or walnut-oil mayonnaise is a good way to get omega-3 EFAs into your family's diet. (With a food processor, it's easy to make any homemade sandwich spread or filler.)

You can get around mayonnaise altogether by making chicken salad with a dressing of oil and tarragon vinegar, then mixing in just enough yogurt to bind it together.

Commercial mustard is all right, but many children don't like it, and it's not suitable for all sandwiches. Try a mild, whole-grain mustard such as Pommery with cold meat or poultry, or a relatively sweet Dijon tarragon mustard with poultry or cold fish. You can also mix tarragon mustard with yogurt and a little oil to make an interesting spread or dip. Use one part mustard to two parts yogurt and a dash of oil, and mix well. It's not necessary to buy the bright yellow hot-dog mustards.

Fillers. This is a good way to use leftover *meat, fish, or poultry.* For color, taste, crunchiness, and vitamins, include vegetables in the sandwich, or separately—sliced tomatoes or green peppers provide vitamins A and C, for instance.

Nut butters make excellent fillers. I'm not happy about peanut butter because of a strange quirk in the way its oils are structured. It has a tendency to raise cholesterol levels, so walnut and almond butters are preferable, although harder to find. Walnuts contain omega-3 EFAs and almonds are rich in magnesium. (See Chapter 10.)

If you do use peanut butter, look for Smuckers, which is free of sugar or corn syrup. Or buy freshly made, pure peanut butter at the health-food store—try it salt-free as well as sugar-free.

To make nut butters, especially peanut butter, more nutritious, mix in sesame butter (tahini) and/or soy flour or ground sunflower seeds. These add protein, zinc, and copper.

To make nut butters more flavorful, add apple butter, chopped dates, or raisins for sweetness. For taste, texture, and vitamins mix in or add to the sandwich such vegetables as shredded carrots (vitamin A), alfalfa sprouts, sliced tomatoes, or sliced green peppers (vitamins A and C).

Hummus, made of mashed chick-peas, makes a good substitute for nut butter. You can use nut butters or hummus every day; for their high magnesium, serve them at least twice a week. You can add flaxseed oil to nut butters to make them moister.

Fish and salads. Squeeze lemon on an individual can of tuna or salmon, or some sardines. Canned salmon is high in vitamin B-12, sardines in calcium, iron, and vitamin D. Both supply some omega-3 EFAs, but not enough, in the canned form, to obviate the need for flaxseed or cod-liver or walnut oil. Canned tuna is rich in niacin and other B vitamins, but read the label for its salt content. Even low-salt brands may have hidden salt; I advise rinsing all canned fish before you use it.

Make chicken, turkey, or tuna fish salads with homemade mayonnaise or tofu (see Chapter 10).

Add sliced tomatoes or sprouts to these sandwiches. Some children like minced olives, but be sure to rinse them off.

Desserts

A piece of fresh fruit is best: send along an apple, pear, peach, quartered orange, or banana. Don't use dried fruits or oatmeal cookies because they leave sugary deposits on the teeth, and most children don't get to brush their teeth after lunch at school. (In fact, sending a toothbrush with lunch is not a bad idea, if she remembers to use it.)

AFTER-SCHOOL SNACK

Children need to eat more than three times a day because they are active and growing. A healthy after-school snack can make an important contribution to your child's diet.

Milk or *yogurt* both make excellent snack foods, although your child shouldn't need more than two cups of milk a day.

Lunch sandwiches also make excellent snacks.

Homemade fast foods will be essential for variety.

- Add chopped *fresh* or *dried fruit* and *nuts* to plain, low-fat yogurt.
- *Mini-pizza:* broil a whole wheat muffin with cheese and tomato; or *pocket-pizza:* fill a whole wheat pita with mozzarella and tomato, and bake five minutes in a 350° F. oven.
- *Granola bars* (see Chapter 10 for recipe).
- *Crackers or chips with spread or dip.* Avoid such standard fare as corn or potato chips; they're loaded with heat-damaged, partially hydrogenated vegetable oils and salt, as are most crackers, for that matter. Ry-Krisp and Ideal, and the Scandinavian crisp breads (Wasa, Kavli) are made without oil. If you can find commercial tacos or tortillas without added oil, they can make good chips. Just bake the tortillas until crisp (see Chapter 10). Use nut butters on crackers, make Mexican bean or tofu dip, or season yogurt with dill or chopped chives. Add flaxseed oil to nut butters to turn them into dips, or add yogurt to sesame butter (see Chapter 10).
- *Yogurt or tofu smoothies* (see Chapter 10) make great snacks; you can also freeze them to make pops.
- *Homemade, low-sugar, oatmeal-sesame-raisin cookies* (see Chapter 10).
- *Frozen nut-fruit balls,* made with chopped dried fruit, nuts, and seeds (see Chapter 10).

SUPPER

I can't emphasize enough the importance of making this a family affair, even if only one parent can be there. Eat at the kitchen or dining-room table, and talk to each other. Don't watch TV or read. Eating should be, deliberately and consciously, a complete experience, not something you do on the run, or while doing something else. But if you don't set the example yourself, your child will never learn the pleasure of a relaxed meal in the company of loved family.

If your child has had a high-protein breakfast, a nutritious lunch, and a wholesome after-school snack, you don't need to fix a big dinner. A light supper is fine: soup, salad, and bread may be all she needs.

Many families eat most of their daily protein at dinner, but, as we have seen, this is a mistake, especially for children. Now is the time for carbohydrates.

Carbohydrates

Starches. Most children love mashed potatoes, but you can be more inventive than that. Serve brown rice, whole-grain breads, kasha, or whole wheat spaghetti or noodles. Add kasha to cooked noodles; your child will love it.

Soups. Both hot and cold soups make excellent supper items. Cuisinart has an excellent pressure cooker that doesn't have to be cooled down and in which you can make the most complicated soups in just 30 minutes. To chop vegetables, a food processor saves more time.

Vegetables. Serve a variety of vegetables, and keep the different colors in mind for different minerals and vitamins. Try to have at least one baked or steamed green vegetable plus one orange or yellow vegetable. You can also stir-fry vegetables.

For topping, instead of using high-fat butter or margarine, squeeze a fresh lemon over your vegetables, or make my basic flaxseed-oil or walnut-oil and vinegar dressing. You can add herbs and/or minced garlic to the dressing. Grated cheddar or Parmesan cheese makes an excellent topping.

Experiment with various combinations of vegetables, or make a whole meal combining different textures and colors. That artful and versatile bean food, tofu, seems made to be stir-fried with a variety of vegetables.

Protein

You will eat some protein at supper.

Beans. Serve them twice a week, if possible. You can combine them with pasta and sauce, or rice, or fish or poultry. In addition to protein, beans provide magnesium, soluble fiber, minerals, and lectins, natural chemicals that stimulate the immune response of the white blood cells in the intestines.

Seafood. Serve two or three times a week. Shellfish and scaled fish are low in saturated fats and supply omega-3 EFAs and essential minerals. My bouillabaisse recipe is a whole meal in a bowl. (See Chapter 10.)

Meat. Liver is rich in vitamin A, zinc, iron, and the very important B vitamin, folic acid. Your child needs all of these nutrients to keep building a strong immune system. For that reason, I sometimes recommend eating liver at least once a week.

Beef, lamb, pork, and veal are high in saturated fat, so don't serve this group more than twice a week. (If possible, get organic beef, now available in a few supermarkets.) It may take a while to lose the craving for—or the habit of—eating red meat more frequently, but eventually you will find you enjoy other sources of protein.

Poultry. The best way to serve chicken or turkey is roasted. Buy a fresh small turkey or a Bell and Evans chicken from your butcher. Fresh poultry tastes better and is likely to be healthier than its battery-raised, thawed supermarket counterpart. To roast poultry, clean the cavity and rub the inside with a sliver of fresh garlic. (If you like the taste of garlic, leave two or three cloves in the cavity.) Rub the outside of the bird with fresh paprika. (Buy the best Hungarian paprika and keep it in the refrigerator.) Roast in a low-heat oven. Set the bird on a rack so that the fat drips down into the pan.

Another method for chicken is to brown it first to keep in the flavor and juices, then cook it with a cup of chicken broth or VegeBase for thirty minutes in a Cuisinart Pressure Cooker/Steamer. This saves time and retains flavor, minerals, and vitamins. However you cook poultry, though, remove the fat-loaded skin before serving.

Dessert

It is traditional after dinner, but it's here that many parents' best intentions go awry. Yet desserts can be nutritious as well as delicious. I generally avoid honey—nutritionally, it's not much better than sugar. I rely on fruit for sweetness and vitamin C, yogurt or tofu for calcium, and nuts and seeds for other minerals.

Many of the snack foods listed above—yogurt with chopped fruit, or homemade granola bars, smoothies, oatmeal cookies, or frozen nut balls—make excellent desserts. So do yogurt or tofu pudding or freezer pops, low-sugar fruit-nut pies and spice cakes with optional creamy yogurt or tofu toppings. These are all easy to prepare, and you can make them ahead of time in batches. (See Chapter 10.)

Baked apples are a snap and fill the house with a wonderful aroma. In baking, some starch turns to sugar, making the apples sweeter. You can simply bake washed, cored apples for an hour in a low oven with a little cinnamon. Baste them in their own juice as they cook. If you like, add a few unsulfured raisins and a tablespoon of homemade granola in the core cavity.

Fresh or dried fruit (preferably without preservatives) is the only preparation-free, commercially available dessert that's not loaded with anti-nutrients.

HOLIDAY AND PARTY FOOD

Any of the snacks and desserts are fine for parties. Popcorn is all right, but nutritionally limited—you can add nourishment by sprinkling hot popcorn with grated Parmesan.

Pretzels are better than chips because there's no added fat, but they're basically just white flour and salt, and supply almost nothing nutritive.

Halloween is a real challenge: make it into a celebration of the autumn harvest season with our Pumpkin Pie (see recipe in Chapter 10), apples, warm cider with cinnamon sticks, pumpkin seeds, and walnuts. Halloween Pumpkin Cookies and Granola Bars (see recipes) are good for goblins and other trick-or-treaters.

Christmas is a holiday for sweet, moist, nutritious spice cakes and fruit breads, with lots of goodies mixed in. For Easter, try fruit and nut balls wrapped in colored foil instead of jelly beans and chocolate. (See Chapter 10.)

Encourage your child to help prepare such holiday treats in advance; you'll both enjoy the sharing and the creative fun. (See other suggestions in Chapter 8.)

Omega-3 essential fatty acids (EFAs) help maintain your child's immune system in top form, protect her against cancer and heart disease later in life, and ensure that her nervous system functions properly. So it is vital that you give your child omega-3s in some form every day. The easiest way is to give her 1 tablespoon flax-seed oil or 1 teaspoon cod-liver oil each day. She can take it straight, like medicine, just before a meal or juice, or you can mix it into her food or juice. (Drink quickly, because juice and oil soon separate.)

If you notice that your child is excessively thirsty, or if she has dry skin or dull, lifeless hair, she may have an EFA deficiency. For a full discussion of how to deal with this, see page 16.

Vitamins C and E and magnesium are key supplements for a properly regulated immune system. All are completely safe. A healthy child following my basic meal plan needs no nutritional supplement as a rule, except for flaxseed oil or the substitutes for it I have suggested. If there is a strong family history of allergy, or if the child has problems with allergies, infections, or behavior, these supplements may be added to a healthy diet.

Vitamins C and E

Five hundred milligrams of vitamin C and 100 international units of vitamin E daily provide children with greater antioxidant protection than good food alone can give them. These two vitamins are especially indicated for children in urban or industrial areas who are exposed to considerable air pollution.[1]

Magnesium

Growing children need 6 milligrams of magnesium per pound of body weight every day. This amounts to about 240 milligrams a day for a small five-year-old and 600 milligrams a day for a growing twelve-year-old. These figures, calculated by the American expert Dr. Mildred Seelig, executive director of the American College of Nutrition, and her European counterpart, Dr. Jean Durlach, chairman of the Society for Development of Research on Magnesium, are greater than current RDAs. Seventy percent of

American children consume less than two-thirds the RDA in their food each day, so they are getting an even smaller fraction of their real need.

Magnesium has a subtle but very important effect on her immune system: it is among the most important of the co-factor vitamins and minerals that help the body metabolize EFAs to make prostaglandins. And prostaglandins, you may recall from Chapter 1, are the chemicals that regulate the immune system as well as many other systems in the body. For instance, magnesium deficiency causes the body to release more histamine, which increases the severity of allergic symptoms such as congestion, coughing, and shortness of breath.

The best food sources for this important mineral are nuts, nut butters such as almond or peanut butter, seeds, vegetables, and seafood.

Magnesium deficiency can also be caused by increased excretion of magnesium in the urine. High intakes of salt (sodium), sugar, fats, protein, phosphorus, or vitamin D all increase magnesium excretion. So do stress and physical exercise. If your child is very athletic she will need a plentiful supply of high-magnesium foods.

If your child is athletic and/or has been eating a typical American diet, high in salt, sugar, fats, and the other anti-nutrients, she may also need a supplement. If she has allergies, she definitely does.

Typical symptoms of mild magnesium deficiency include:

Irritability: restlessness, poor sleeping habits, hyperactivity
fatigue
muscle spasm: twitches, abdominal pain, headaches, or bed-wetting
creepy-crawly feeling on the skin: older children who are able to verbalize their symptoms may describe this as a pins-and-needles sensation
grinding the teeth at night

If your child has any of these symptoms, you can find out whether it's caused by magnesium deficiency by a simple test: Give her an oral magnesium supplement for four weeks and see whether the symptom or symptoms improve in that time. This can be a much

better way to determine magnesium deficiency than any laboratory measure now available. You will soon know if the dose is too
high because your child will develop diarrhea. If she does, just
reduce the dose. (If your child has a kidney problem, consult your
physician before using any magnesium supplement. Children with
kidney problems can develop too high a level of magnesium in
their blood.)

When I saw six-year-old Betsy, she was a nervous child who slept
poorly and was constipated. Almost every day she complained of
abdominal pain. Her reflexes were hyperactive: when I tapped the
skin over her facial nerve, it twitched. (This is called Chvostek's
sign.) Betsy wasn't getting much magnesium in her diet, and her
symptoms suggested deficiency to me. When I prescribed three
magnesium chloride tablets a day, her abdominal pains, irritability, and constipation disappeared, and she began to sleep better.

Which Magnesium Supplement to Use. Magnesium comes
in a bewildering variety of forms. All magnesium (and all other
mineral) supplements contain the mineral attached to something
else such as an oxide, chloride, citrate, gluconate, orotate, aspartate, amino acid chelate. A 500-milligram magnesium oxide pill
contains about 200 milligrams magnesium and 300 milligrams
oxide—each element weighs about the same. Magnesium orotate,
on the other hand, supplies only about 30 milligrams of magnesium in a 500-milligram pill, because the orotate makes up 470
milligrams. A true amino acid chelate of magnesium supplies 30
to 50 milligrams of magnesium in a 500-milligram tablet. If it
claims to supply more, it's not a true chelate; it's a mixture of
magnesium oxide and amino acids that isn't any better than plain
magnesium oxide.

Magnesium oxide is safe and can be effective, but it usually
comes in a big, chalky tablet that is hard to swallow. So-called
amino acid chelates, including magnesium aspartate, are expensive and seldom worth the money because they usually contain
primarily magnesium oxide but cost much more.

Magnesium citrate is a good magnesium source if it's given
in a sublaxative dose. (Magnesium citrate is a common laxative,
but a sublaxative dose won't have that effect.) One tablespoon
daily of magnesium citrate can correct a magnesium deficiency

for just pennies. Unfortunately, most magnesium citrate liquids contain artificial flavor, sugar, and/or Sorbitol. Pure magnesium citrate capsules are available in some pharmacies and can be bought by mail from Hickey Chemists, Ltd., 888 Second Avenue, New York, N.Y. 10017.

Magnesium chloride is an excellent source of magnesium; the chloride enhances its absorption. A good source is Slow-Mag, enteric-coated magnesium chloride tablets. The coating decreases gastric irritation. Give your child three tablets a day. Taken at bedtime, magnesium can enhance sleep. (If you can't find Slow-Mag in your pharmacy or health-food store, order it from the manufacturer: Health Care Technologies, Inc., Indianapolis, Ind. 46202.)

Not recommended. Antacids such as Maalox and Mylanta contain magnesium but they also contain aluminum, a toxic metal. Magnesium carbonate, from dolomite, is often not well-absorbed, and dolomite is often contaminated with lead.

Calcium

School-age children who dislike, or don't tolerate, dairy products tend to become calcium deficient. This can be a serious problem because it produces brittle bones, and may also produce symptoms very similar to those produced by magnesium deficiency, such as muscle spasm and irritability. In fact, calcium complements magnesium in its calming, muscle-relaxing effects.

Your child only needs about two cups of milk or yogurt a day to avoid a deficiency: 1 cup of milk supplies 288 milligrams; 1 cup of yogurt supplies 174 milligrams.

Other calcium-rich foods are almond butter, bean soup, and tortillas. For a more complete list of calcium-rich foods, see page 101.

If your child is not eating or drinking two cups of milk or yogurt every day, *and* if she's not eating lots of nondairy calcium-rich foods such as fish with bones (canned salmon, sardines, and herring), "bitter-tasting" collard and mustard greens, tofu, shellfish, or nuts, I recommend 600 milligrams of a calcium supplement daily. I don't recommend more than that amount because too much calcium interferes with vitamin D metabolism and with your child's ability to absorb zinc and iron.

Recommended forms. Calcium carbonate from oyster shells is one of the cheapest forms of calcium. It is best absorbed with stomach acid, so always give it to your child with food. Chewable calcium carbonate wafers, with no sugar or coloring added, are available at health-food stores: 600 milligrams daily.

Calcium citrate is best if your child has allergies, because allergies are sometimes associated with a decrease in the production of the stomach acid needed to absorb calcium carbonate. Give her two to three tablets a day.

Not recommended. Calcium carbonate from bone meal or dolomite, both of which can be contaminated with lead. Tums, which contain sugar and talc (talc has been shown to promote tumors in animals).

Zinc

This element continues to be one of your child's most important nutrients. It is a key co-factor mineral, helping the body metabolize EFAs, and it is also an important antioxidant, protecting white blood cells while they protect your child. Zinc deficiency impairs immune function and predisposes a child to many different kinds of infection. It can also impair growth.

Strenuous exercise, high-protein diets, and allergies increase the loss of zinc from the body. Diets too high in iron and calcium can block the body's absorption of zinc. Mild zinc deficiency, like mild magnesium deficiency, is very hard to test. Dr. Ananda Prasad, one of the world's foremost authorities on zinc, says that the best test for zinc deficiency is functional. Since one sign of zinc deficiency is white spots on the fingernails, if your child has such spots an easy functional test would be to give your child a zinc supplement and see whether they disappear.

Jon was a seven-year-old boy with a history of bed-wetting, colds, and behavioral problems. He didn't sleep well, his attention span was poor, and he was hyperactive. He also had dry skin and his fingernails were marked with white spots. His parents were giving him cod-liver oil and vitamin C, with no observable improvement.

When I measured the level of vitamin A in Jon's blood, I found that despite the cod-liver oil it was low. Because the body needs zinc to use vitamin A, and because of the white spots on his nails, I suspected that Jon was zinc deficient. I used a new, very accurate and nontraumatic test of zinc status: a measurement of zinc in sweat. It confirmed the deficiency. Since Jon couldn't swallow pills, I recommended 10-milligram zinc lozenges. Jon sucked on one lozenge a day. Over the next two months he developed fewer colds and fewer white spots and his skin became shinier. His blood vitamin A levels increased to normal.

Recommended forms. Because excessive zinc supplementation lowers the body's levels of such other key minerals as iron, copper, selenium, and manganese, and because high zinc levels can also elevate cholesterol, I don't recommend zinc supplementation lightly. When it does seem necessary, I recommend that zinc be taken as part of a multimineral preparation such as Bronson Insurance Formula or Mineral Formula (Bronson Pharmaceuticals, La Canada, Calif. 91011-0628), available only by mail, or Basic Preventive, Jr., from Advanced Medical Nutrition, Inc., Hayward, Calif.

Zinc lozenges are effective when a child can't swallow pills, but she should take the companion minerals listed below. Zinc lozenges also have a local anti-viral effect and are useful in treating viral (non-strep) sore throats. A child can suck on up to six a day for three or four days.

Zinc lozenges made to my specifications can be obtained from Freeda Vitamins, 36 East 41 Street, New York, N.Y. 10016.

Unless your child is under supervision by a physician with a knowledge of nutrition, *her daily dose should not be more than 10 milligrams.* If white spots on her nails persist after two months of this supplement, she either needs a higher dose or her nail problem is caused by something other than zinc deficiency.

Minerals That Go with Zinc. To prevent depletion of other minerals because of zinc supplementation, your child's multimineral supplement should also include:

copper	1 mg	
manganese	10 mg	(manganese is poorly absorbed from supplements after the first six months of life)
selenium	75 mcg	
chromium	200 mcg	
molybdenum	200 mcg	

Chromium protects against heart disease, diabetes, and hypoglycemia. Chromium supplements have normalized the blood sugar of diabetics and hypoglycemics. Molybdenum helps the body use sulfur, a substance found in all tissue, which is critical to normal immune function and to antioxidant activity.

Many people seem to be "allergic" to sulfites, which are frequently added even to fresh foods as preservatives. Dr. Carl Pfeiffer, of the Brain-Bio Center, Princeton, New Jersey, has found that such people usually have a molybdenum deficiency and are thus unable to break down sulfites properly. Instead of an allergy, they have a metabolism problem.

Chromium is found in whole grains and in brewer's yeast; molybdenum in meats, whole grains, legumes, and leafy vegetables.

Iodine

Although essential for normal thyroid functioning, in excess iodine can cause acne and contribute to the development of a thyroid inflammation called thyroiditis. If your child eats seafood, she won't need iodine or kelp supplements. If she doesn't eat seafood, a pinch of powdered kelp or 60 micrograms of iodine daily in a multivitamin will be enough.

Iron

Also a key mineral, it is crucial both to brain functioning and in keeping up a high volume of red blood cells to carry oxygen to the body's tissues. In addition to anemia, with its attendant listlessness, iron deficiency can affect a child's capacity to think and remember, and so affect her school performance.

A good screening test for iron deficiency is a check by a physician on the level of ferritin—a protein that stores iron—in the blood. Children with low ferritin levels, while they may not be anemic, tend not to function well intellectually compared to children with normal levels.[2]

Alice, age six, was not exactly in wonderland when I saw her. She was tired all the time, and far behind the other children in school. When I investigated her eating habits, I discovered that she drank about a quart of milk a day, in addition to yogurt, cheese, and ice cream. She was borderline anemic with a very low blood ferritin level, and her red blood cells were somewhat small and pale.

I advised her parents to cut down on the dairy products Alice ate and drank so that she would be hungry enough for other foods. Ice cream and cheese were the first to go since they had the least to offer. Milk and yogurt were restricted to between-meal snacks.

In addition to remedying Alice's iron deficiency, I wanted to change her eating habits so the problem wouldn't crop up again. But she didn't like the taste of meat and she didn't like to chew. I advised her mother to prepare soft, flavorful stews with bits of meat or clams or oysters.

I also suggested a teaspoon of blackstrap molasses in Alice's breakfast cereal to provide iron and calcium. But blackstrap molasses is an acquired taste, and Alice wouldn't acquire it. So I prescribed a chewable multivitamin with iron, plus a chewable vitamin C—both twice a day with meals for maximum absorption. Within a month, Alice was like a new girl.

Iron is best obtained from foods, in combination with other minerals. Meat, poultry, and shellfish are the best sources. Eggs contain some iron, but not in a form readily available to the body. Vitamin C increases iron absorption, so it's a good idea to serve vitamin C–rich fruits and vegetables with eggs, meat, and iron-fortified cereal.

TO GET 15 MG OF IRON A DAY FROM FOOD

(serve 2 portions from this list: 3 mg each)

Tuna	1 cup
Turkey, dark	¼ lb
Red meat	¼ lb
Pumpkin seeds	2½ Tb
Almonds	⅓ cup
Sunflower seeds	⅓ cup
Pinto beans	¼ cup
Soy or kidney beans	½ cup
Lima beans	½ cup
Spinach	½ cup
Peas	1 cup
Tomato juice	1 cup

3 portions from this list: about 1 mg each

Egg	1
Chicken	¼ lb
Salmon	½ cup
Oatmeal	¾ cup
Whole wheat muffin	1
Shredded wheat biscuit	1
Brown rice	1 cup
Tofu	2 oz
Lentils	¼ cup
Winter squash	½ cup
Broccoli	1 cup
Potato (medium)	1
Peanuts	¼ cup
Sesame seeds	⅓ cup
Brazil nuts	¼ cup
Hazel nuts	¼ cup
Shredded coconut	¼ cup

Iron Supplements. I don't recommend an iron supplement for school-age children who aren't actually iron-deficient. Unneeded iron blocks the absorption of zinc, manganese, and molybdenum, undermining the immune system.

If your child is iron deficient, the best way to deal with it is to feed her foods rich in iron: red meat three or more times a week for a month, seafood stew twice a week, chile con carne (beans with ground or chopped meat) often. Give her tomatoes, broccoli, or citrus fruits with meat so that the vitamin C can increase the amount of iron she absorbs.

Or you can use a supplement. I recommend Kovitonic, a liquid iron made by Freeda Vitamins. She should have about 15 milligrams of iron a day. It's best to give an iron supplement with food, but not with bran, which prevents absorption. Unless she eats a high-bran cereal for breakfast, give her iron at breakfast and supper. After three months, have her ferritin level tested again.

FIGHTING THE JUNK-FOOD JUNKIES

Junk food is ubiquitous in our culture, and sooner or later your child is going to want to eat it. She'll be exposed to it on TV, at the supermarket, at friends' houses—even, sadly, at school. Increasingly, she'll be spending most of her days away from home, and will have to deal with the temptations of junk food on her own. What can you do? Plenty.

- Don't bring junk food into the house. If your child asks for it, explain carefully and patiently that you love her and for that reason will only bring healthy food into the house.

- Limit her TV viewing to a few hours on weekends. Television advertising is particularly difficult for a child to resist because it conveys seductive images and a lot of subliminal messages. You can explain to her that TV ads exaggerate because they are designed to sell what they're advertising.

- Provide lots of colorful, chewy, healthful snacks such as carrot sticks, zucchini, cucumber, cherry tomatoes, cauliflower and broccoli florets, and green and red pepper chunks with yogurt or nut butter dip, oatmeal cookies, popcorn sprinkled with grated cheese, chick-peas, whole wheat muffins, minipizzas, tortillas and tacos, low-fat yogurt with fresh fruit, smoothies, granola bars, fruit-and-nut balls, and fruit freezer pops (see Chapter 10). Your child and her friends can help make many of these snacks, which is half the fun.

- Eat a healthy diet yourself. Your example can work for or against you. If you tell your child not to eat what you eat, she's going to wonder about the double standard. And she's not going to believe you if you tell her that adults are immune from the harmful effects of bad food. If you snack on nacho potato chips, she's not going to see anything wrong with them no matter what you tell her.

- If you're eating the same kind of healthy diet you expect her to eat, start explaining what's behind it. Tell her a healthy body needs protein, vitamins, minerals, and the right oils for peak performance, and that these things come from vegetables, fruits, whole grains, seafood, poultry, and so forth—not from sugar and fat. She can understand that sugar and fat just fill her up without giving her body any of the nutrients it needs. Stress the importance of good food for the attributes that are important to her: Good food will make her feel good and look good. It will help her to be smart and strong and athletic, and help keep her from getting sick.

- Assert your rights at school: visit the school to find out what your child is being encouraged to eat there. Visit the lunchroom during lunch hour. Check for candy and soft-drink machines. If the situation is not what you would want, have a frank talk with the teacher and the principal. Join the PTA and campaign for healthier lunches and snacks. (In addition, as we discussed on pp. 149–151, you should send your child to school with a brown-bag lunch.)
- To help her cope with the different eating patterns of other families, tell her that, while other families have other ideas about what to eat, you expect the parents of other children to respect your ideas about what is best for your children. A child who believes that you love her and want her to eat right so that she can become strong and successful in school will be more likely to follow your guidance even when you're out of sight. You're still the major authority figure in her life, so when she's with friends whose parents may offer foods you would not allow her to have, she'll be able to say "no, thank-you" easily and courteously because she wants to please you.
- Discuss nutrition with the parents of your child's playmates. You may find that, while many of them agree with you in principle, they feel they have no control over their children much of the time, or just give in to social pressure. Explain your position to these parents and seek some common ground. Obviously, if your child eats meals at another house, you expect her to eat what she's served. Explain your thoughts about the worst anti-nutrients: soda, chips, candy, and sweet junk foods. Request that these items not be offered to your child during after-school visits.

If your child is well-fed by you all week, a weekend party at which she's fed soda, gooey cake, and ice cream by someone else's parents won't harm her. Good friends are as important as good food, maybe more so. Explain to your child that by eating well all week, she is, in fact, being fortified against the effects of weekend indulgence at those sleep-overs and parties that mean so much to her.

HOW TO USE NUTRITION TO COPE WITH THE SPECIAL PROBLEMS OF SCHOOL-AGE CHILDREN

OBESITY

My basic diet plan doesn't provide the empty calories that can lead to obesity, but you may have a problem if your child is very inactive, if she craves sweets and eats junk food away from home, or—an unlikely occurrence—if she eats too much of the healthy food you serve her. Since obesity is a major problem among school-age children today, how can you nip the problem in the bud? You need a dual approach: through activity and through food.

You also need to realize that children want to be like their parents, so you *must* set a good example. It's crucial that you eat the same kind of healthy foods you expect your child to eat. Stress how important it is to be healthy and to grow up strong and resistant to illness. If you are changing your eating habits, let your child know how much better you feel. Take the lead in physical activity and include her and the rest of the family. You may have to change your own life-style, but it will be well worth it.

At seven, Mack was a bit chubby and a poor eater. He was a sedentary child who liked very few foods. At school, he would trade his bag lunch for cookies and candy. In fact, he wasn't much different from his mother.

I realized that there wasn't any point in trying to change Mack's behavior; this was a family problem. I enlisted his mother in the project. She had to confront her own style of eating and her own sedentary habits, but as she began to make changes she enlisted Mack as a buddy. They exercised together and began to plan healthy menus together. Mack started helping with the cooking.

Within a few months, the family's habits were very different, and Mack was a changed child. He began to feel good about himself not only because he looked and felt better but because he was not the object of a prescription for change. He was an agent in a positive family process.

Activity

Some children are born more active than others. If your child is relatively inactive by nature, you can help by creating opportunities for physical activity, by being active yourself, and by helping your child find some area of movement that pleases her. At school or the Y she may be able to choose swimming, basketball, volleyball, punchball, or games classes. If you live in the north, skating and skiing will be available in the winter. Folk dancing is good exercise.

Sharing activity can provide motivation for both of you. The whole family can take brisk walks, ride bikes, go swimming or folk-dancing, play softball, touch football, or volleyball, or ski or skate together. You can follow an aerobic movement show on TV with your child, or dance to music. Your child should engage in some brisk activity every day, and it won't hurt you, either.

Of course, all these suggestions are useful for active children and parents, too. Sharing activities is a great way to share love and good feelings.

Be sure to praise your child for all her physical activity. This is crucial.

Food

In addition to all the tips I give above, under Fighting the Junk-Food Junkies, there are some more useful tips for dealing with an overweight child.

Never force her to eat or tell her to "clean her plate." Don't bargain with her, either, and never use sweets or dessert as a reward or treat. Saying, "You have to finish all your food to get dessert," will just make dessert seem like the best part of the meal. In fact, encourage her to stop eating when she feels full. That way, she'll learn not to overeat. Encourage her to eat slowly by putting down her fork between bites and chewing deliberately. If she's a fast eater, this may take time to master, but the rewards are better digestion and a more relaxed meal. Do the same thing yourself.

Call foods "healthful" and "unhealthful" rather than "fattening" and "nonfattening." Tell her you don't eat junk foods because your body is not a garbage dump. Praise her when she chooses healthy foods.

Encourage her to eat the lower-calorie healthy foods—fish, poultry, rice, potatoes, vegetables, and fresh fruit—rather than the higher-calorie items such as nuts, seeds, dried fruits, fruit juices, cheese, and milk.

Don't display tempting items such as cookies, nuts, or chips in your home. Don't keep a glass cookie jar out on an open shelf, for instance. Don't keep candy at all.

If your child craves sugary or salty foods, encourage her to notice the varied tastes of the well-prepared foods you serve. Sweet and salt are not necessarily acquired tastes, but eating lots of sweet or salty foods numbs the palate to more delicate and subtle flavors. The less she eats sweets, the less she will crave them. Gradually, the nutritious, naturally sweet desserts you learn to make will come to seem sweet enough to satisfy her—and you.

Above all, *don't* encourage dieting. Weight depends on over-all eating patterns and levels of activity—and crash diets can be harmful. Anorexia and bulimia (self-starvation and binge eating followed by vomiting) are major problems among adolescent girls today, and the eating habits and skewed self-images that lead to these problems are being formed in childhood.

Overweight children tend to have very poor self-images. If your child is overweight, one of the most important things you can do is to help her develop a better self-image. *Never* call attention to her weight; instead, talk to her about how she feels about herself. Point out her positive traits: is she funny, friendly, cooperative, caring, sharing, affectionate, inventive, loyal, a good student, a good listener, musical, clever, good with her hands, fun to take on trips and share adventures with, athletic, artistic?

Like Mack, she will feel better if you involve her in the nutritional changes you make: discuss the nutritional value of foods with her so she can help you plan menus. Get her involved in preparing food, too.

ALLERGIES

If your child has chronically itchy skin, eyes, or anus; frequent skin rashes; or dark circles under her eyes, she may have an allergy. Snoring and nasal congestion that seems to be a reaction to cats, dogs, plants, or such indoor spaces as basements or barns are also symptoms. So are abdominal pains, headaches, chronic fatigue, asthma, and some behavioral problems.

Allergies are helped by my basic diet, including flaxseed oil and a magnesium supplement. In young children, headaches and abdominal pain particularly suggest a magnesium deficiency; I would give them 3 milligrams per pound of body weight every day as a supplement. If that doesn't work, double the dose.

Allergic children often become less allergic if they supplement their diets with the co-factor nutrients for proper EFA metabolism and with antioxidants to decrease allergic inflammation:

vitamin A	5,000 mg daily (as beta-carotene)
vitamin B-6	10 mg daily
vitamin E	100 units daily
vitamin C	500 mg daily
zinc	10 mg daily
copper	1 mg daily
manganese	10 mg daily
selenium	75 mcg daily

Supplements supplying these amounts are listed on page 161.

Food

To detect a food allergy, follow these steps, focusing on two specific items:

Milk. As the most common food allergen, this is the place to start. If your child drinks a lot of milk or eats a lot of cheese or yogurt, try the five-day elimination diet. Eliminate from your child's diet *all* milk, butter, cream, cheese, yogurt, ice cream, and any foods containing milk, milk solids, or milk derivatives. Read all labels carefully to look for whey or sodium caseinate, derived from the milk protein casein. (For more on milk-elimination diets, see p. 86.)

Yeast. If your child begins to show *some* improvement on the five-day milk-elimination diet, stay with it and begin to investigate yeast. If there is no improvement, drop the milk-free diet and check out yeast. A child who has had antibiotics more than once a year, who has *any type* of allergy, who has behavioral problems of any kind, or who develops behavioral problems *after* antibiotic treatment might have a yeast sensitization problem.

As I explained in Chapter 6, antibiotics destroy the good intestinal bacteria that normally kill yeast. When a child becomes sensitive or allergic to this yeast overgrowth (*Candida albicans* is the species of yeast involved), the sensitivity can extend to other types of yeast and to molds, and can intensify *any* allergic problems, from asthma to hyperactivity. A yeast-elimination diet can help identify the culprit.

It's important to limit natural sugar, including dried fruits and commercial fruit juices. Sugar aggravates a yeast allergy by stimulating yeast growth in the mouth. (As you will see next, dried fruits and commercial fruit juices are full of yeast, too, so you will want to eliminate them.)

To check for an allergy to the yeast and mold found in food, you will have to eliminate many other items from your child's diet. Yeast and mold are found in most cheese and breads and crackers; they are also used as additives in pasta, bread, crackers, and many canned items (including soups, which may contain yeast extract); eliminate these.

Yeast grows naturally on the skins of such fruits and vegetables as peaches, apples, and tomatoes. So products made from them, such as fruit juices, dried fruits, and tomato sauce are all pretty yeasty. Peel fresh fruits and vegetables, and prepare fresh orange or grapefruit juice yourself. Eliminate canned or bottled fruit juices if you haven't already, and fruits (such as berries) that can't be peeled.

Vinegar is made by the action of yeast, and it can be found in pickles, catsup, mustard, mayonnaise, barbecue sauces, and salad dressings. Eliminate all of them.

Vitamins may also contain yeast; make sure your child's are yeast-free.

Malt, another yeast product, is used as a flavoring in many breakfast cereals. Restrict your child to oatmeal, puffed wheat, and puffed rice. Read labels of drinks to be sure malt hasn't been used as a flavoring.

Your child *can* eat meat, poultry, fish, eggs, rice, oats, peeled fresh vegetables and fruit (limit fresh fruit to two pieces a day), and such yeast-free grain products as matzoh and rice crackers.

Keep your child on this diet of "safe foods" for five days. Then reintroduce vinegary foods, dried fruit, bread, commercial fruit juices, and cheese (if dairy is okay) for two days. If your child improves during the five-day elimination and deteriorates when yeasty foods are reintroduced, she may have an allergy to yeast in food.

If the elimination diet helps, keep it up for a while. If it doesn't, or causes too much resistance, you have two choices:

- Consult a physician who works with food allergy. You can obtain a list of such physicians from The Academy of Environmental Medicine, P. O. Box 16106, Denver, Colo. 80216.
- If your child has had lots of antibiotics or you've seen allergies develop or get worse after antibiotics, you can take steps to decrease intestinal yeast growth nutritionally.

On your own, you can restrict artificial and natural sugar: no honey, dried fruit, fruit juice, punch, soda, cake, etc., and no more than two pieces of fruit a day. *Acidophilus,* a bacteria normally found in the large intestine, helps keep down yeast growth there. The best products are milk-free Primeplex from Klaire Laboratories or milk-containing Ultradophilus from Natren: give your child about 1 teaspoon a day.

If your child can swallow pills, you can give her *caprylic acid.* A nonessential fatty acid found in coconut oil, caprylic acid kills yeast when taken internally. Two good preparations, sold in health-food stores and some pharmacies, are Capricin (Professional Specialties) and Caprinex (Murdoch Pharmaceuticals).

Caprylic acid is classified as a nutritional supplement and is extremely safe. Six to twelve capsules must be taken *with food* every day. Because killing yeast can release allergens that at first worsen allergies, I recommend starting with a small amount of caprylic acid and slowly increasing the dose. Start with one capsule of Capricin or Caprinex twice a day (breakfast and supper), and raise the dose per meal by one more capsule every two days to a maximum dose of three to six capsules per meal. Continue the full Capricin dose for two months. If it helps, you'll need further guidance on this problem. Read *The Yeast Connection* by William Crook, M.D.

Asthma

This is one of the most difficult problems that commonly afflict young children; at worst, its effects can be tragic—a crippling loss of breath, even death. Fortunately though, most of the time it can be treated with nutrition and without drugs. If an effective allergy-desensitization technique is used, and as much environmental control as possible is exercised, drug-free treatment is virtually always possible in children.

Here are some guidelines for asthma treatment:

- Put your child on my basic low-sugar healthy diet.
- Flaxseed oil: 1 tablespoon daily
- Magnesium: 3 milligrams per pound of body weight each day
- Eliminate milk and all milk products and derivatives. (Many asthmatics are allergic to milk.) Give her a 600-milligram calcium supplement each day.
- If there is a history of antibiotics or cortisone use (there usually is), check for a yeast problem and treat it as described above, pp. 170–72.
- The following nutritional supplements have been found to play a definite role in asthma:

Fatty acids: High doses of fish oils suppress the formation of leukotrienes, which cause the bronchial tubes to constrict. I recommend 1 tablespoon of cod-liver oil or, better yet, 6 grams of MaxEPA (fish-oil extract capsules) a day.

High doses of vitamin C: About 2 grams a day help to improve the flow of air by dilating the bronchial tubes through an indirect effect on prostaglandin formation, a reduction in histamine levels also occurs.[3]

Vitamin B-6: A study at the world-famous Cleveland Clinic showed that asthmatic patients have difficulty maintaining vitamin B-6 in its active form. A dose of 200 milligrams a day helps these patients.[4]

Vitamin B-12: Low levels of vitamin B-12 have been found in studies of asthmatic children who lacked stomach acid. High doses of B-12 given by daily injection have cured some of the more severe and unresponsive asthmatics, with the best results occurring in children. The dose is 1 milligram twice a day for about six weeks *(Ouch!)*. Fortunately, I have not had to use this method since others often work so well.

COMMON INFECTIONS

Health isn't the absence of disease; it's the ability to overcome it. As they grow up, healthy children catch and get over a number of infections. Because of immunization, few get measles or mumps anymore, but colds and the flu are still common. These are viral infections, and they need no specific treatment. In fact, the worst thing to do is to treat a viral infection with antibiotics— these drugs have absolutely no effect on the virus and they just encourage yeast infections. Aspirin may help lower fever and relieve pain, but it increases the length of viral infections. Fever is actually a protective mechanism, and I would not lower a child's temperature unless it goes over 103° F. or the child is in a lot of pain. (At this age, febrile convulsions are rare.)

At ten, Sam had a stuffed nose and complained about frequent stomachaches and headaches. He said he felt "sick" most of the time. His parents had found that food made him sick, and had put him on a very limited diet that avoided most fruits, dairy products, cereals, and eggs. Despite this diet, though, he was still sick most days.

Right after coming to see me, Sam caught the flu. I recommended that his parents not give him aspirin or Tylenol to suppress his fever, and they let it run its course over several days. When it was over, Sam was completely well—he had no symptoms of allergy at all. He remained in remission for six months.

You can diminish the severity of cold and flu with vitamins C and A in higher-than-nutritional doses: 1,000 to 2,000 milligrams (1 to 2 grams) of vitamin C a day, 10,000 units of vitamin A. These doses can safely be given for two weeks.

The truth is that healthy children benefit from occasional virus infections, and should be allowed to experience them. The exception is a child who has chronic or recurrent colds, frequent sore throats (strep or viral), or asthma. In such children, viral infections further weaken the immune system instead of strengthening it. What they need is immune boosters.

Immune Boosters

If your child catches everything that comes around, I recommend the following in addition to my basic meal plan, flaxseed oil, and magnesium:

Vitamin C. When your child gets a virus, the vitamin C levels in his body drop. School-age children (five to ten) can safely take up to 2,000 milligrams (2 grams) a day. After that, let your child's body fight the virus. When she gets better, taper the vitamin C back down to 500 milligrams a day. Doses of vitamin C in the 1,000- to 3,000-milligram-a-day range enhance immune function in healthy people.[5]

Vitamin A. Carotene, the form of vitamin A found in plants, is an effective antioxidant. Retinol, the form of vitamin A in animal foods, supports the action of your child's killer T-cells. Virus infections deplete a child's vitamin A stores.[6] Administer 10,000 units a day in a capsule, or 1 teaspoon of cod-liver oil a day, or increase her intake of vitamin A from animal sources (liver, eggs, butter), using the guidelines on pages 107–108.

Zinc and Iron. The importance of these minerals for immune function was explained on pages 102–106. Increase the amount of zinc and iron your child gets in food, using the guidelines on pages 103–104, or supplement her diet with the minerals as described on page 105.

Fish Oils. If your child has more than two respiratory infections a year and her skin is dry despite flaxseed oil, she may not be able to use flaxseed oil well as a source of omega-3 EFAs. Try using fish oils. A teaspoonful of old-fashioned Norwegian cod-liver oil for a five-year-old to a tablespoon for a twelve-year-old will serve and will supply plenty of vitamins A and D as well—so cut out the liver supplements.

Alternatively, you can give her fish-oil capsules (MaxEPA or Efamol Marine), 2 to 3 grams per day. The omega-3s in fish oils are chemically different from those in flaxseed oil. They are longer and more unsaturated. In fact, they're the most naturally unsaturated oils that exist. Some children, especially those with allergies, cannot form these extra-unsaturated EFAs well themselves, and need to consume fish oils to compensate.

In Addition

Water. When she's sick, don't force your child to eat, but make sure she drinks plenty of fluids to prevent dehydration; pure water and juice are good, or dilute fruit juice with water.

Yeast. If she's had lots of antibiotics, check out a possible yeast problem. I've described the specific steps for this investigation above, under Allergies.

Allergy. Look for indications of an allergy: itchy skin, eyes, or anus; skin rashes; dark circles under the eyes. Also snoring, nasal congestion related to the environment (the presence of cats or dogs, being in barns or basements, or attending parties) or the season.

HYPERACTIVITY

The most common behavioral problem children at this age have is adjusting to school. In many cases, there may be a comparatively simple reason: often, a child is developmentally immature for the demands of her grade level. This is especially likely to happen to a bright child, whose intellectual development exceeds her chronological age and whose social development lags behind both.

I believe such a child should not be pushed ahead; she may, in fact, greatly benefit from being allowed to repeat a year so that her social development can catch up to that of her peers. The Gesell Institute in New Haven has devised a developmental scale to assess youngsters. If you need help in evaluating whether or not your child should be allowed to repeat kindergarten or first grade, check with your school district; they may have a Gesell expert on staff. Or contact the institute. In any case, don't let a feeling of false pride keep you from making a decision to let your child repeat a year. Some of the happiest, best-adjusted kids I know were immature in first grade, repeated it, and have made steady, successful progress since.

Then there are the children whose problems involve irritability, short attention spans, and generally difficult behavior. These children are often called *hyperactive* or are considered to be suffering from an *attention-deficit disorder*. Until the 1970s, such children were often called bad, lazy, or stupid. Now it is recognized that they need help—and, increasingly, that their problems may be biochemical in origin. Behavioral difficulties of this type can have a psychological or social background, such as the stress of a divorce. But when a troubled child's home is stable, my experience has shown that nutrition and food allergy often play important roles.

For instance, Peter couldn't sit still in class, and he constantly whistled or made popping noises. The minute he felt frustrated or was rebuked, he would burst into tears. He wet his bed every night, and he had a terrible self-image. Although he loved milk and drank a quart a day, he was thirsty all the time. The dark circles under his eyes suggested an allergy.

I suspected Peter's problem was milk, one of the most potent food allergens in young children, so I recommended that he go for five days without milk, butter, cream cheese, yogurt, ice cream, or any other foods containing milk, milk solids, or milk derivatives. (Milk derivatives include whey and casein. Casein is often added to packaged foods as sodium caseinate.) Instead, he got water and diluted juice.

Peter didn't like this change very much, and he was no more attentive in school. But he stopped making popping noises, and he stopped bed-wetting. These were significant changes, clues that we were on the right track toward finding the ultimate culprit. Peter actually had many allergies and deficiencies, as usual, of magnesium and EFAs.

To help your hyperactive child, you'll need to do a little detective work. Ask the following questions:
• Is her diet healthy, or does she eat lots of sugar and junk foods? To be a sugar sleuth, you must read the ingredients on prepared foods. Most of the sugar eaten by kids is not table sugar; it is hidden in food by the manufacturer. The following are all fundamentally sugar: *dextrose, corn sweetener, corn syrup, fructose,* and *honey.*

Don't use foods that include any of these among the first five ingredients.

- Is she very thirsty?
- Does she regularly wet her bed?
- Does she have dry hair or skin?
- Has she had antibiotics recently, or has she had several antibiotic treatments in her life?
- Are there any foods, such as milk or vinegar, that she seems to crave?
- Does she have allergic symptoms such as puffy eyes, runny nose, cough, itchy skin?
- Is there a family history of allergy?

If the answer to any of these questions is yes, it's time to begin work. The three critical nutritional areas you will investigate are *EFAs, magnesium,* and *food allergies.*

EFAs

First, eliminate junk food from your child's diet. Follow the diet plan in this chapter for a low-sugar, nutritionally rich diet supplemented with flaxseed oil, 1 tablespoon a day (or substitute 1 teaspoon of cod-liver oil or 2 tablespoons of walnut oil), to provide omega-3 EFAs. Get food-grade flaxseed oil. It should be almost tasteless; if it tastes at all bitter, it is rancid; throw it out. (See Chapter 1 for a full discussion of EFAs and flaxseed oil.)

If your child has a specific EFA deficiency, she may be excessively thirsty, her skin may be dry, and her hair may be dull and lifeless. If flaxseed or walnut or cod-liver oil is the key to correcting her deficiency, you will know after a month; her thirst will be back to normal, her skin will be smoother, her hair silkier and more lustrous.

If, on the other hand, your child becomes *thirstier* with the flaxseed or walnut or cod-liver oil at any point from a few days to a month, the deficiency may involve omega-6 EFAs. Such children are usually hyperactive *boys;* they may have enzymes that are so sensitive to omega-3 EFAs that the small amount provided by the usual American diet is actually enough for them. Stop the oil you are using and substitute safflower oil: 1 tablespoon a day. Or, better still, give your child evening primrose oil, two to three 500-milligram capsules a day, or two to three 250-milligram capsules of black currant oil.

Be careful when you buy primrose oil; it's so expensive that bogus cut-rate brands have begun to appear. They are useless. I recommend sticking with Efamol brand. One distributor is Nature's Way (Murdoch Pharmaceuticals, Inc.).

If primrose or black currant oil is going to help at all for different specific problems, you should expect to see results as follows:
- Excessive thirst, restless sleep: a return to normal patterns within seventy-two hours.
- Bed-wetting: expect a change for the better within a week.
- Other behavioral problems will take about a month—again, *if the oil is going to help at all.*
- Dry skin and hair will take about two weeks.

Should you raise the dosage if your child shows no improvement, or improves in only one area? I'm often asked this question, and my advice is that if three 500-milligram capsules of primrose oil or three 250-milligram capsules of black currant oil a day produce a beneficial change in *any* area, it means that the oil is having some effect. Therefore, *don't* raise the dosage—just give the oil more time to work. Too much of these oils has been known actually to *reverse* the beneficial effect.

But if you see absolutely no change in *any* area after three weeks, then raise the dose by one pill a day, give that dosage for seven days, then add one more pill for seven days, and continue adding one pill a week until your child is taking a *maximum* of six pills a day. If there is still no effect, go on to the next step.

Magnesium

The next step is to give your child a magnesium supplement. Give 3 milligrams per pound per day as Slow-Mag (see p. 159)—this will take two to six pills a day—or as magnesium citrate liquid—1 to 2 tablespoons daily or capsules (one to three capsules daily). Do this *in addition to* the primrose or flaxseed oil; the two may have an additive effect.

Calcium

If your child drinks *less* than two 8-ounce glasses of milk a day, or eats its equivalent in yogurt, add a calcium supplement according to the instructions on p. 101.

Not recommended. Megavitamin therapy is usually not at all helpful with hyperactive children; in fact, it often makes their behavior worse. The B-vitamins are especially tricky: Some children are allergic to the yeast used in making most B-complex tablets or capsules. Others simply have adverse reactions to the B-vitamins themselves. I've found that hyperactive children are generally also hypersensitive; they overreact to stimuli, whether chemical, sensory, or emotional. In fact, they are living examples of the unity of mind and body. Instead of pouring more supplements into their bodies, now is the time to do some allergy detective work.

Food Allergies

It is well-established that allergies to foods and food additives, and to inhaled chemicals and mold spores, play a role in hyperactivity. (For a fuller discussion of the scientific evidence for this, see Chapter 6, pp. 133–41) Once you've tested for the effects of EFAs and added magnesium to your child's diet, some food trials are in order. (Follow the procedure outlined on pp. 86–87.)

Jethro was a child whose behavioral problems stemmed entirely from a yeast overgrowth as a result of antibiotics. At eight he wasn't a bad-natured child, but his frenetic behavior drove his mother crazy. He had been a normal baby until he had a couple of ear infections. Both responded to antibiotics, but after the second one, and two courses of antibiotics, Jethro at eighteen months became a changed child. Instead of the bright, alert child he had been, he became spacey during the day and restless and wakeful at night. For a while, his parents thought he would outgrow this behavior; instead, it became worse. Jethro began to wet his bed. He had a hard time getting to sleep and was hard to get up in the morning. He seemed intolerant of changes and had problems adjusting to school. Because of his poor record, he was being evaluated for a special-education program.

We laid out a strategy that included:

* A balanced, low-sugar diet
* Acidophilus: ½ teaspoon Primeplex twice a day with food (It tastes quite pleasant.)
* Twelve Capricin pills a day. (For a description of Capricin, see p. 172.)

Jethro started on one pill each at breakfast and supper, and increased slowly to six pills with each of those meals.

During the first four to six weeks of this treatment, Jethro's behavior gradually improved. His school performance went from consistently poor to variable—he now had good days as well as bad ones, and the bad ones weren't as bad as they had been.

At this point, we put Jethro on the yeast and mold elimination diet, and it worked wonders. In fact, he became a new child—or, perhaps, just the child he was becoming before he was sidetracked by his ear infections and antibiotics.

The earlier you treat problems such as hyperactivity or asthma with sound nutrition, the better the results of the treatment will be and the more cooperation you are likely to get from your child. Adolescents are particularly willful and rebellious—their special needs are described in the next chapter.

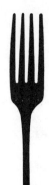

Ages Thirteen to Seventeen: Keeping Your Teenager in Top Health

8

Adolescence is hard on parents and adolescents alike. You've been feeding your child a healthy diet, and his play has given him plenty of exercise. But now he may skip lunch at school to hang out with the other kids at McDonald's or Pizza Hut. He's not interested in vegetables: given a choice, he'll go for anything sweet and sugary or fried and fatty. He is *certainly* not willing to go to school with a nutritious sandwich in a brown bag. Unless he goes out for school sports, he's probably not getting a lot of exercise, either. As soon as he's old enough, he'll drive rather than walk or ride his bike.

Throughout his adolescence, he'll have to make difficult choices concerning cigarettes, alcohol, drugs, sex, and ethics (whether or not he should be honest about doing homework or in dealing with other people, both his peers and adults, including you). He wants very much to believe in your values, but at his age example is more crucial than ever. If you skip breakfast, why shouldn't he? If you can't take the time for regular exercise, why should he? If you have a drink to relax at the end of the day, why shouldn't he? You can, of course, forbid him to drink and exhort him to exercise, but in the absence of your positive example he's bound to discount your words. What's more, you'll be undermining one of the most precious things in your relationship, his belief in you.

Your teenager's self-interest provides you with a couple of points in favor of good nutrition: He's starting to care a great deal about his looks. He's worried about his skin, his hair, and his physique. The best road to a lean body, clear skin, lustrous hair, and shining eyes is, of course, through nutrition and exercise. If your teenager is an athlete, a little clear information should help convince him that good nutrition is essential for top-notch performance. In fact, a teenager is well able to absorb the basic nutritional information in the first chapter of this book, and in this chapter as well.

Your teenager is under a lot of pressure: His hormones are creating immense physiological changes to which he must adjust while also heeding pressure to succeed academically, socially, and perhaps athletically. Peer pressures are especially intense at this age, and the choices he faces are more than difficult; they have potentially dangerous consequences, from addiction to AIDS. In the pages that follow, I will offer guidelines to help you cope with one important area that affects what happens to him in all the other aspects of his life: nutrition. If he is getting the best nutrition you can give him, he will be in a better position to cope with the stresses of the rest of his life. All his systems, including his immune system, will be "go."

It should go without saying that your teenager needs lots of love and attention. He may not always be able to ask for it, so sharpen your sensitivity and learn to be there before you are called.

THE SPECIAL NUTRITIONAL NEEDS OF ADOLESCENTS

A teenager's tendency to forget that such things as fresh vegetables exist makes the usual teen diet much too low in folic acid, vitamin A, and essential fatty acids—all crucial to the health of his immune system. What's more, sexual development in boys increases their need for zinc, which is concentrated in semen. The zinc that is lost in ejaculation must be replaced through nutrition.

Rising levels of estrogen in girls produce changes in the way their bodies handle vitamin B-6 and magnesium. As a result, they need more of both.

But if your teenage son or daughter is eating a lot of lunches and snacks with the group at Burger King, what are you going to do? Well, first of all, it's not the end of the world. It would be worse if he or she didn't have any friends. Concentrate on the meals you can control—breakfast, supper, and (sometimes) after-school snacks. And give him some basic supplements. Although I don't advocate a broad program of preventive nutritional supplementation for younger children, I do think it is worthwhile for adolescents.

DIETARY ESSENTIALS FOR YOUR ADOLESCENT

Your teenager needs a moderate amount of protein, a lot of fiber and minerals, and very little fat, sugar, and salt. Many studies in the last few years have linked fats to cancer, heart disease, high blood pressure, arthritis, and multiple sclerosis. Marbled red meats and pork and such high-fat dairy products as whole milk and cheese should be served seldom and in small amounts.

A diet high in salt contributes to hypertension and strokes. Sugar supplies calories without nutrients and contributes to obesity and several vitamin and mineral deficiencies.

THE TRUTH ABOUT CALCIUM AND STRONG BONES
Or Why a Pepsi or Coke Is the Worst Thing for Your Teenage Daughter

Osteoporosis is a major health problem among American women. Most begin losing bone density at menopause, but whether or not they actually develop osteoporosis depends to a great extent on how dense their bones are before that. A woman has about twenty years to develop dense bones—from puberty to her early thirties. After thirty-five, it's too late to build bone density; she can only try to prevent bone loss.

Two factors help build dense bones in adolescence: *exercise* and *diet*. Weight-bearing activities such as walking, running, or tennis, which put pressure on bones, especially the legs and spine, stimulate the formation of new bone tissue. Swimming, which puts no pressure on bones, does not help prevent osteoporosis.

Walking is an excellent exercise, available to everybody. I encourage regular family walks—at least a half hour a day. It's a good way to spend time with your kids and a healthy habit.

Nutrition for building healthy bones starts with calcium, the major bone mineral. But calcium alone is not enough; the right amounts of several key co-factor nutrients are needed: protein, phosphorus, magnesium, manganese, copper, silica, and vitamins A and D.

The first step in forming new bone is the laying down of a soft, rubbery protein called *bone matrix*. Crystals of calcium, phosphorus, and magnesium, deposited on the matrix, make it hard and rigid. The rate at which calcium is deposited depends on many nutritional and hormonal factors, the most important of which is the level of calcium in the blood. This in turn depends partly on the amount of calcium absorbed from the intestine, and *that* reflects both the amount of calcium in the diet and the amount of vitamin D in the body.

Because osteoporosis is such a big problem, American women are generally advised to take a lot of calcium and vitamin D. Alas, this advice is quite irrational. To understand why, we have to understand the intricate mechanisms that control the absorption and use of calcium in the body.

The level of calcium in your teenager's blood is tightly controlled by a hormone called *parathyroid hormone* (PTH), which is produced by the four tiny parathyroid glands that sit on the thyroid gland. Among other things, PTH activates vitamin D. Vitamin D is different from all other vitamins. In fact, it isn't really a vitamin at all; it's a hormone produced by the skin when it is exposed to sunlight. And to be of any use, it must be activated by PTH. Active vitamin D, or *calcitriol*, increases the rate at which calcium is absorbed from food in the intestine.

When the level of calcium in the blood falls, the parathyroid glands secrete more PTH, which in turn converts more vitamin D into calcitriol. The calcitriol increases the amount of calcium that's absorbed from food.

When the level of calcium in the blood goes up, the parathyroid glands stop secreting PTH, and the body stops making calcitriol for a while. If a person eats a lot of calcium or starts taking calcium pills, blood calcium goes up, so PTH secretion drops and calcitriol levels fall. The result is that *less* calcium is absorbed even though there is more available in the intestines!

So if you consume only a moderate amount of calcium rather than a megadose, you'll absorb a higher percentage of it. Howard Rasmussen of Yale University, one of the world's leading calcium experts, points out that the chief effect of increasing calcium intake from 600 milligrams a day (considered low in the United States) to 1,200 milligrams a day (considered desirable in the United States) is that calcitriol production falls, and so, therefore, does the percentage of calcium absorbed from the intestine. The extra calcium just goes out in the stool. (This does *not* hold true, though, for a diet that is seriously *deficient* in calcium. *Six hundred milligrams a day are essential.*)

THE CRUCIAL CALCIUM CO-FACTOR NUTRIENTS

Rasmussen's observations are only valid if the calcium-PTH-calcitriol regulatory mechanism is working. It generally works less well in the elderly, but in adolescents it should work very well *if* their diets are also rich in the calcium co-factor nutrients: magnesium, phosphorus, vitamin A, and essential fatty acids (EFAs).

Magnesium. Magnesium is essential for the release and activity of PTH; both are impaired by magnesium deficiency.

Phosphorus. A two-edged sword, it is essential for laying down bone, but in excess it blocks both the secretion of PTH by the parathyroids and the absorption of calcium and magnesium from the intestines.

The American diet is marginally low in magnesium and excessively high in phosphorus. Phosphorus is found in rich supply in meat and in preservatives. Most important for adolescents, it is used to keep nearly all soft drinks bubbly. There is nothing worse for the bones of a teenage girl than Coke or Pepsi.

Vitamin A and EFAs. Both are required to enable calcitriol to do its important work in the intestinal tract.

Magnesium, copper, and *manganese* help move calcium from the blood into the bones. Unfortunately, teenagers' diets are often deficient in these minerals.

Some Food Sources of Calcium Co-Factor Minerals

Food sources of these important bone minerals are our old friends: seafood, beans, vegetables, whole grains, nuts, and seeds. Silica is mostly found in water; the nutritional herb horsetail *(Equisetum)* is also a rich source. Horsetail tea would be a great substitute for soft drinks. If a teaspoon of honey were needed for a teenager to accept it, the trade-off would be worth it. Other foods for healthy bones include:

FOOD	MAGNESIUM (mg)	COPPER (mg)	MANGANESE (mg)
Cod, mackerel, bluefish, ¼ lb	30	1.5	trace
Brown rice, 1 cup	45	trace	3.2
Oatmeal, 1 cup	75	trace	1.5
Brazil nuts, ½ cup	175	1.0	2.0
Almonds, ½ cup	140	0.4	1.3
Sesame seeds, ¼ cup	104	0.9	0.6
Walnuts, ½ cup	95	0.5	0.7
Tofu, ¼ lb	112	0.8	1.0
Spinach, 1 cup, cooked	100	0.3	1.4

A MEAL PLAN FOR ADOLESCENTS

Your teenager needs a variety of nutritious foods: fish, poultry, lean meat, eggs, low-fat milk products, fresh and dried fruits, nuts, seeds, beans, vegetables, all types of grains (rice, corn, oats, wheat, and so on).

At home, you will want to avoid serving some foods altogether:

Fatty Foods. Fat contains over twice as many calories per gram as starch or protein, and when it is used for frying, as for potato chips, it is usually loaded with toxic breakdown products.

In addition, most high-fat foods contain the kinds of fat that interfere with the body's ability to absorb calcium and magnesium and to metabolize EFAs. You will want to eliminate fried foods completely, also bacon, hot dogs, lunch meats, commercial pizza, hard cheeses, virtually every variety of commercial chips, cream, ice cream, and margarine.

Sugar. High-sugar foods include many breakfast cereals, commercial baked goods, all candies, catsup. Read the label on every container or package of manufactured food. If sugar, corn syrup, dextrose, or fructose is one of the first few ingredients, don't buy it. And since most manufactured foods are high in salt as well as sugar, you'll kill two birds with one stone.

Phosphates. Preservatives and soft drinks are high in added phosphates. Limit beef to twice a week, tops.

Here's a food plan that will enable you to feed your teenager nutritious, interesting, and convenient breakfasts, after-school snacks, and suppers.

BREAKFASTS

Citrus juice or cut-up orange slices—plus any of the following:

Cereal. For a sweet, crunchy, high-fiber, mineral-rich, and easy-to-cook cereal, mix equal parts of rolled oats and oat bran, and add small amounts of chopped walnuts, sesame and sunflower seeds, raisins, and/or chopped dates. Add milk or yogurt if desired.

Homemade Granola or Muesli (see Chapter 10).

Nutritious Sesame Waffles (see Chapter 10).

Blueberry whole wheat pancakes (see Chapter 10).

Toasted low-sugar Bran Muffins (see Chapter 10). Serve with apple or almond butter or low-fat cottage cheese and chopped fruit.

Poached or boiled egg and whole-grain toast.

BAG LUNCHES FOR SCHOOL

If you can persuade your teenager to take a bag lunch, I suggest you follow the suggestions in the previous chapter, including my recommendations for types of bread.

AFTER-SCHOOL SNACKS

- Keep pancakes or waffles in the freezer. Heat and serve with applesauce or fruit purée. If you need to use canned fruit on occasion, be sure to rinse off the syrup.
- Pita bread pizza. Fill a whole wheat pita pocket with low-fat mozzarella and fresh vegetables. Bake for five to ten minutes.
- Unsalted mixed nuts.
- Mexican Bean Dip served with carrot or celery sticks, Tortilla Chips (see Chapter 10) or crisp bread. Cook in batches, freeze, and thaw as needed. Do *not* use commercial corn chips, which are high in fat. Instead, break tortillas into smaller pieces and toast.
- High-protein Granola Bars (see Chapter 10).
- Soup. You can make it for immediate consumption or freeze batches for later use. Serve with whole-grain toast, crisp bread, or bran muffin. Good choices for batch cooking: bean, lentil, creamy tomato, clam chowder.

SUPPERS

Supper is usually too large and too full of protein these days. I favor lighter, low-protein suppers—one dish plus bread and salad. You can use the suppers in Chapter 7; if you have more than one child you will want to prepare the same supper for both. But teenagers are sometimes willing to be more adventurous than younger children; try the following on yours. See recipes in Chapter 10 for Seafood Ratatouille, stir-fried vegetables and tofu, Lentil and Barley Stew, or Tofu-Ricotta Lasagna.

DESSERTS

Check the recipe section in Chapter 10 for nutritious, low-sugar desserts. Fresh fruit is always good.

PARTIES

If you serve nutritious party foods that teenagers can enjoy, you will serve your own cause by showing your children and their friends that good food doesn't need to be boring. Don't call atten-

tion to the fact that the party treats are healthy, though. They are
sweet, crunchy, and tasty; they don't need an explanation.

Some party food ideas (check Chapter 10 for these and other
ideas):

Tofu Custard
Spice Cake (carrot or apple) with a special frosting
Oatmeal cookies (no extra sugar)
Apple cinnamon pie
Fresh popcorn; liven the taste by sprinkling with Parmesan
Fruit-nut cocktails
Smoothies
Pumpkin cake
Baked apples
Carrot sticks and peanut butter
Celery sticks stuffed with low-fat cottage cheese or hoop cheese
    (available fresh in some cheese stores)
Skewered fruit and chunks of Cheddar cheese
Trail mix
Homemade, no-sugar banana or blueberry sherbet
Frozen banana pops and crunchies
Yogurt freezer pops

Holiday Party Treats

Halloween. Fresh popcorn, trail mix, oatmeal cookies, and
small apples fit nicely in plastic bags for give-aways. At home, you
can also serve frozen cider pops, baked apples, pumpkin cake, nut
balls, a favorite dessert, or whole wheat pizza.

Christmas or Hanukkah. Try Tofu Custard and Spice Cake.

Easter. Hard-boiled Easter eggs, Ambrosia (for sweetness
and bright colors). Freeze homemade sherbet in bunny and chick
molds. Fill Easter baskets with homemade sweets wrapped in
colored foil or paper. Mix chopped dried fruit, nuts, and peanut
butter, cover with coconut.

NUTRITIONAL SUPPLEMENTS

My work with several thousand patients has convinced me that a
broad-based program of nutritional supplementation is a good

idea for adolescents and adults alike. Although my diet plan is designed to supply a complete range of nutrients, adolescents have special needs. They are in a period of rapid growth and emotional stress, and they may also be performing strenuous exercise. Inevitably, they are eating some junk food, full of anti-nutrients. For all these reasons, nutritional supplements are a good idea.

Here is a list of the supplements I recommend. The most important—because they are most likely to be deficient—are asterisked.

Vitamins

B VITAMINS

Thiamin (B-1)	10 mg
Riboflavin (B-2)	15 mg
Niacinamide (B-3)	100 mg
*Pyridoxine (B-6)	25 mg
Pantothenic acid	100 mg
*Folic acid	400 mcg

I don't routinely use large doses of B vitamins. In addition to being unnecessary, they can make acne worse. Also I don't like to include vitamin B-12 in multivitamin pills because a mixture of vitamin B-12, C, B, and copper in the stomach can change B-12 into a harmful substance called a B-12 analogue that can actually interfere with the action of B-12 in the body.

*Vitamin A (as beta carotene)	15,000 units

Beta-carotene has no known toxicity. The body changes it into active vitamin A, or retinol, at a controlled rate. I sometimes use retinol supplements; the indications for retinol are described later in this chapter.

*Vitamin C	1,000 mg
*Vitamin E	400 units

Vitamin C and vitamin E are antioxidants. They protect the body from the toxic effects of free radicals, chemicals that can damage tissues and cells. Free radicals are found in heat-damaged oils such as those used to fry or deep-fry any food. They can also be created when white blood cells burn off such poisons as air pollutants (the formaldehyde in new carpets and new clothes, fresh paint, solvents and cleaning solutions, car exhaust, Epoxy cement, for example) or heavy metals that contaminate drinking water (cadmium and lead from water pipes, the mercury that leaches out of a fresh dental filling).

Minerals

*Magnesium	300–500 mg
*Zinc	15 mg
*Copper	1 mg
*Selenium	100 mcg
Manganese	10 mg
*Chromium	400 mcg
Molybdenum	400 mcg

The manganese dose may appear high compared to the RDA, but manganese in pills is very poorly absorbed, and 10 milligrams is quite safe. The only danger with oral manganese supplements occurs in newborn infants, because they absorb it so readily.

I don't include iodine for the same reasons I don't like large doses of B vitamins—it is usually unnecessary, and can make acne worse.

I also omit iron because it blocks absorption of zinc, copper, and manganese. Iron deficiency can be a problem with teenage girls. They should be checked periodically, and if their serum ferritin is low or falling, then they should take a separate iron supplement: 20 milligrams chelated iron twice daily with food and 500 milligrams of vitamin C to enhance absorption. They should take this for three months or until the ferritin becomes normal.

Chromium and molybdenum are trace minerals, often lacking in the U.S. diet. Chromium plays a role in stabilizing blood sugar. Chromium deficiency may contribute to diabetes and hypoglycemia.

EFAs

*Flaxseed Oil	1 Tb daily or
Cod-Liver Oil	1 teaspoon daily or
Walnut Oil	2 Tb daily

HOW TO COPE WITH YOUR TEENAGER'S HEALTH PROBLEMS

Many of the health problems to which adolescents are prone are partly or completely rooted in nutritional imbalances or inadequacies. Acne, obesity, bulimia, fatigue, menstrual cramps, mood and behavioral problems, headaches, mononucleosis, irritable bowel syndrome, and sore throats can all be helped, and some can be cured, through proper nutrition. The bonus is that a healthy diet may clear up more than one problem—headaches may disappear along with acne, for instance. Good nutrition restores the body's systems to good working order, while medical treatment merely deals with a specific symptom.

ACNE

Acne is the single most common problem affecting teenagers. It is *always* caused by a biochemical imbalance in the body, and several reports show an association with a modern Western diet.[1] For that reason, proper nutrition can help alleviate it and may prevent it.

At twelve, Lewis had oily facial skin with blackheads and a bumper crop of pimples; at fourteen, he developed serious acne. He told me that none of the lotions his friends used worked for him. When a dermatologist prescribed the antibiotic tetracycline, his mother refused to let him give it to Lewis. She told me that she had also had acne as a teenager and had developed a serious yeast allergy from the same antibiotic.

I explained that acne is caused by an overproduction of *sebum,* an oil produced by oil glands in the skin under the influence of hormones. When the oil is thick, it may become trapped in the pores, producing whiteheads. When sebum is exposed to air, it darkens, creating blackheads.

Skin bacteria break down the sebum into irritating fatty acids that produce red pimples and cysts. The usual medical treatment involves antibiotics to inhibit the action of these bacteria and lotions to peel off the top layer of skin and clear the pores.

Male hormones and stress can stimulate sebum production, as can deficiencies of zinc, vitamin A, and vitamin B-6 or too much iodine. Allergic reactions to foods also increase sebum flow in some adolescents. In my experience, the old notion that rich foods, sweets, chocolate, and fats cause acne is valid in about 50 percent of the cases.

I realized that Lewis needed to revamp his diet. I outlined a diet rich in vegetables and low in sweets, pastries, and fatty foods. Lewis had no trouble dropping such fatty foods as bacon, fried foods, and chocolate cakes, but he wouldn't or couldn't let go of his pizza and ice cream obsessions.

Lewis was taking a high-potency multivitamin. I had him stop it immediately. Most people think megadoses of vitamins help clear up acne, but some B vitamins can make it worse. I find that vitamins A and B-6 and zinc, without other Bs, usually work best.

But Lewis had normal blood levels of A and B-6, and normal levels of zinc in his hair and sweat.

I decided to explore the role of stress. While his diet changes had improved his acne, it invariably flared up again whenever he was under stress. At such times, he also ate large quantities of ice cream. I wondered whether a milk allergy might be another culprit. I persuaded Lewis to stop eating or drinking milk, and all foods containing milk or milk derivatives for a full week. At the end of the week he could pig out on milk and ice cream for a day.

The first part of this treatment is *elimination,* when we see whether eliminating a specific food or group of foods improves an allergic condition. The second part, the pig-out, is the *challenge,* when we see whether adding a specific food back to the diet worsens the allergy. To work well, the elimination must be complete. Lewis had to forego milk, cheese, cream, ice cream, yogurt, butter, and bread and cakes made with milk, milk solids, or whey. He had to watch out for two milk proteins—casein, sometimes seen on labels as sodium caseinate, and lactalbumin—commonly used as food additives. Caseinate is used in margarine and non-dairy creamers.

Lewis's skin didn't clear up much on the milk elimination diet, but when he challenged it by pigging out on milk, cheese, and ice cream, his whole face broke out in pimples. Subsequently, several weeks of a balanced diet that eliminated all milk products helped clear his skin up. That did it: Lewis was now convinced that milk products, including his beloved ice cream, were involved in making his acne worse.

But he would still break out from stress—every test at school gave him polka dots. I had to conclude that although the dietary changes had helped, they couldn't completely clear up his condition. I decided it was time to see whether nutritional supplements would make any difference.

In my experience, the very best test for a nutritional need is simply to see how the body responds to a supplement. Would Lewis's stress acne respond to zinc? I suspected a daily dose of 20 milligrams would work—and it did. But I was reluctant to give him zinc alone, because it can induce other mineral deficiencies. So I switched to a multi*mineral* without iodine that provided the following daily doses: 20 milligrams of zinc, 1 milligram of copper, 100 micrograms of selenium, 10 milligrams of manganese, and 200 micrograms of chromium.

EFA supplements help acne, too. Many adolescents with facial acne have dry skin on their legs. Flaxseed and cod-liver oil can help to shift the balance, drying their faces and oiling their legs.

A Regimen for Acne

Here are the things I advise my patients to do for acne:

Follow my basic low-sugar, low-fat diet
Take 1 tablespoon flaxseed oil or 1 teaspoon cod-liver oil daily
Take 10,000 units vitamin A daily
Take 20 milligrams zinc daily
Take 50 milligrams vitamin B-6—*not B complex*—daily

If there is no improvement after three weeks, eliminate *all* milk and milk products for two weeks. That means your teen should avoid milk, butter, cream, cheese, yogurt, ice cream, non-dairy creamers, margarine, and any baked goods made with milk, milk solids, or whey.

Sometimes higher doses of zinc and vitamin A are needed, but they should *only* be administered under the supervision of a nutritionist or nutritional physician. Studies of nutritional supplementation for acne have yielded the following results:

Vitamin B-6, 50 milligrams a day previous to menses, diminishes premenstrual acne flare.[2] *Vitamin A,* 100,000 IU a day plus *vitamin E* 800 IU, induces relief from acne within a few weeks. Maintenance on lower doses is effective.[3] *Zinc* in doses of 90 milligrams to 150 milligrams a day is as effective as antibiotics.[4]

EATING DISORDERS

Obesity

This is the number-one concern of adolescents, particularly girls. It's a threat to health and can be a threat to a teenager's self-esteem. Most people would say the cure is obvious: stop overeating. But eating too much is not usually the problem: The basic cause of obesity is probably lack of exercise. The *second* cause—and this may surprise you—is malnutrition. Or perhaps it would be better to call it undereating.

Studies show that many obese children do not eat more than other children; in fact, many of them eat less. But fat children are much less active than their thinner friends. They play fewer games and compete in fewer sports, they sit more than they stand, they rarely jump around, and they walk when other children run. In swimming pools, they have been photographed standing and talking!

Television in the home is a major contributor to the increase in obesity in children and adults.[5] TV viewing should be strictly regulated or it soon gets out of hand. It is too easy for your teen to come home from school, flop down on the couch, turn on the TV, and watch it mindlessly. Kids in front of the TV sometimes seem to sink into a comalike state.

I suggest that neither meals nor snacks be served in front of the TV. I also suggest no weeknight viewing except for school assignments and special events. For this reason, I am against separate TVs in bedrooms or the kitchen. Daytime viewing on weekends should also be cut out.

Instead, encourage your teenager to get involved in some

kind of after-school and weekend sports program. If he's not on a school team, there may be community or Y teams, swimming programs, or dance classes. If your teen has not yet had his growth spurt and is too small to play regularly for school teams, help him find a sport he enjoys and can play well.

If you want your teenager to be active, you will have to become active yourself. You can jog or play tennis or racquetball with your teenager, and the whole family can ride bikes and play touch football or volleyball. Long walks or weekend hikes are first-rate exercise, too.

Nutritional Density: Giving the Body What It Needs. Even though they eat fewer calories, Americans today weigh more than their grandparents did. Why? We are less active than our forebears, and the foods we eat actually contain *fewer nutrients per calorie* than the foods our ancestors ate. We eat polished grains, for example.

The nutritional value per calorie is called *nutrient density.*[6] Lean meats, eggs, milk, vegetables, nuts, seeds, poultry, and seafood all have a high nutrient density—loads of vitamins, minerals, and essential amino and fatty acids for each calorie. Sugar, foods in which the main ingredients are sugar and/or hydrogenated oils, and foods made with heat-damaged fats or refined flour products have a very low nutrient density.

So two children might eat exactly the same number of calories, but the one on a diet of high-nutrient-density foods will be well nourished, while the one eating low-nutrient-density foods will be malnourished—and very possibly obese.

Why Crash Diets Don't Work. Dieting often makes the situation worse. When adolescents go on low-calorie diets, they eat much less of certain vital nutrients than they need; they become more malnourished. When they stop dieting, they go back to high-calorie but low-nutrient-density foods. The result is that they gain all the weight back, and they are still malnourished. When they go on another crash diet to lose the weight they have regained, they invariably lose less weight than they did the last time.

An interesting study with obese rats confirms the fact that each new crash diet results in less weight loss: Genetically obese rats were placed on low-calorie diets and lost weight. When they were then allowed to eat as much as they wanted, they gained weight. As these cycles continued, each time they were dieted they lost less weight than they had the time before, while each time they were fed as much as they wanted, they gained more weight than the time before. *The result was that at the end of each recurrent diet they were actually fatter than rats that had never dieted.* This happened even though they didn't eat more calories than the rats that had never dieted. Dieting actually slowed down their metabolic rates.

I strongly believe that the answer to adolescent obesity is not simply cutting calories. If overweight teens are going to lose weight permanently they will have to become more physically active and begin eating high-nutrient-density foods.

I first saw Rebecca when she was twelve. Her parents were both overweight, and she had never been particularly thin. But she had no serious problem until she began to menstruate at ten. After that, she began to gain weight, although she was eating just as she always had. The only change was in her activity; she had become much less physically active.

Becky was upset about the way she looked, and she became self-conscious and shy. She didn't have enough discipline to diet, though, and that ultimately proved to be her salvation.

I started by analyzing Becky's and the family's eating patterns. Breakfast, generally cold cereal and milk, was rushed; there never seemed to be enough time to prepare a nourishing meal and eat it. Becky took her lunch to school, but she often didn't like it and drank a carton of milk instead. After school she felt starved and would eat a cheese sandwich, another glass of milk, and, often, a few cookies. At supper, she usually ate meat, potatoes, and two vegetables, plus bread and butter and another glass of milk. The family didn't eat dessert, but in the evening Becky would watch TV and eat some cookies or cheese and crackers and have another glass of milk before going to bed.

Becky's major problem seemed to be her sedentary life-style, which involved her family as well. I recommended that instead of TV-watching in the evening, the family go for a walk, or do calisthenics together; I suggested they might even search out a nearby Y or community center swim program. Exercising together would both make them more active and get them involved in doing things as a family.

The second problem was that Becky wasn't eating enough high-density food. Luckily, she wasn't a big junk-food eater, either. Most of her calories came from milk, cheese, and white flour. (In fact, I suspected a milk allergy might be the cause of her lethargy and postnasal drip.)

Finally, Becky ate too many of her calories late in the day or just before bedtime. As a result, she wasn't hungry in the mornings, and felt she could get by on a light breakfast and virtually no lunch. But by the time she got home from school she was hungry and ate a cheese sandwich because it was quick and easy.

I recommended the following for Becky:

No snacking after supper
A big, nutritious breakfast
A nutritious, brown-bag lunch at school (see Chapter 10 for breakfast and lunch recipe suggestions).
Only two glasses of milk a day
No cheese, white-flour bread, or cookies in the house
Only high-nutrient-density snack foods in the house

Becky's interest in losing weight motivated her to follow my basic nutritional program, which is not designed as a low-calorie weight-loss program. Over a period of several months, Becky slimmed down considerably. She had more energy, and became much more physically active.

Bulimia

One of several serious eating disorders traceable to malnutrition caused by dieting, bulimia is on the increase among teenage girls. It shows itself in a pattern of compulsive binge eating, followed by self-induced vomiting or the use of laxatives to remove the food quickly from the body.

Bulimia usually starts after a period of extreme dieting, and may also follow a period of anorexia. Sometimes it seems to the teen to be an easy way to control weight. Soon, she (bulimia affects very few boys) becomes compulsive about that control and, paradoxically, her binge/purge cycle becomes uncontrollable.

Bulimics are often depressed, and some experts recommend psychotherapy. But Stephanie Dalvitt-McPhillips, a therapist who suffered from both anorexia and bulimia as a teenager, has developed a different method to use with teens who haven't been helped by therapy.[7]

Dalvitt-McPhillips observed that episodes of bingeing always seemed to be preceded by crash diets of fewer than 1,200 calories a day. In a controlled study of 215 bulimic students, she was able to produce rapid and permanent remission by having them consume a high-nutrient-density diet of at least 1,400 calories a day, supplemented with a multivitamin-mineral tablet. The 200 extra calories a day were enough to prevent binges, and none of her subjects relapsed during the next five years.

Despite their binge / purge cycles, all the young women were slightly overweight when they started the treatment program. On 200 extra calories of high-nutrient-density foods a day, they all lost weight.

Dalvitt-McPhillips's study appears to prove two important contentions:

- It's not how much you eat, but *what* you eat that determines what you'll weigh.
- Bulimia is not only psychological in origin; it is a biochemical disturbance that can be triggered by a crash diet.

The weight-conscious adolescent has to learn that the route to permanent weight control is through sound nutritional habits. Teens who eat lots of vegetables, seafood, and whole grains, and very little sugar, fat, and white flour, will be slim without counting calories.

MENSTRUAL CRAMPS

These are caused by an overproduction of certain prostaglandins, the chemicals that are the end product of EFA metabolism and that regulate every system in the body, including the immune system. The medical treatment is aspirin, or drugs such as Advil, which inhibit prostaglandin synthesis.

But drugs treat only the symptoms; the real cause of menstrual cramps is usually a deficiency of omega-3 EFAs. Magnesium deficiency can make the cramps worse. *I have never seen a case of menstrual cramps that did not respond to EFAs and magnesium.*

I recommend the following:
- Follow my basic low-fat diet plan.
- For omega-3 EFAs, supplement with 1 tablespoon of flaxseed oil daily. Even better might be MaxEPA fish-oil extract, 2 to 6 grams a day. Since too much oil could worsen an acne condition, I always go for the lowest dose that will be effective.
- Supplement with magnesium, about 3 milligrams per pound of body weight. This is often extremely helpful.

RESPIRATORY INFECTIONS, SORE THROATS, COLDS, AND FLU

Some children hardly ever get these irritating illnesses, while others are plagued by them. An occasional respiratory infection is normal at any age, and a healthy event in childhood. Most are caused by viruses, and in those cases antibiotics are not helpful; in fact, they may even be harmful. Although in this age group some respiratory infections—strep throat, bronchitis, and pneumonia—may be caused by bacteria, most cases of bronchitis are viral in origin and don't warrant antibiotics. (Bacterial infections of the middle ear and sinuses may occur also. Fever and localized ear or facial pain are usually present.)

When antibiotics *are* used, there is almost *never* a reason to use anything but the old standbys: penicillin or erythromycin. I am appalled at the cavalier use of new broad-spectrum, superpowerful antibiotics such as Amoxicillin or Keflex for simple respiratory infections. Their use encourages the growth of resistant organisms. They kill off health-promoting bacteria, especially in the intestines, encouraging an overgrowth of undesirable organisms, especially yeast. This is a *major* factor in promoting allergy. *It is no accident that the most allergic generation in history has been raised on antibiotics.* Several times a week I see a new patient whose allergies appeared or became much worse after a course of antibiotics.

Antiyeast Treatment to Accompany Antibiotics

If your teenager has to take an antibiotic, I strongly urge the following concomitant steps to prevent yeast overgrowth:
- *Acidophilus powder or pills.* My first choices are ½ teaspoon Primeplex (Klaire Laboratories) twice a day while on the antibi-

otic and for two weeks afterward or the same amount of Ultradophilus (Natren).

• If your doctor will cooperate, 1 million units (two tablets) Nystatin tablets (prescription required) four times a day while on
the antibiotic and for one week afterward. Nystatin should be
taken on an empty stomach. It is not absorbed from the intestine and works as a kind of intestinal antiseptic against yeast.
Its only side effect is possible intestinal irritation.

Over-the-counter additions to or substitutes for Nystatin
are:

Garlic oil. I recommend Arizona Natural Garlic capsules, three with each meal. These are sold in health-food
stores. The garlic is released in the intestine, so there is no
breath odor.

Caprylic acid. A derivative of coconut oil that kills
yeast. Two good brands are Capricin (Probiologic) and Caprinex (Nature's Way). The dose is three to six tablets twice
a day with food. Caprylic acid will upset some stomachs, just
as Nystatin can.

Stay away from such combination products as Yeast
Fighters; they contain a little caprylic acid but they are generally ineffective.

Vitamins C and A

Some nutritional supplements are helpful in fighting *acute*
viral infections. For the child with occasional mild infections (less
than three a year) I recommend rest, chicken soup, and TLC. For
severe infections with fever, lots of aches, and/or uncomfortable
congestion, I find short megadose therapy with vitamins A and C
helpful.

Vitamin C and Immunity. Almost two decades ago, Linus
Pauling began making controversial claims about the value of
large doses of vitamin C in preventing and treating the common
cold and other illnesses. He has since argued that adults should
take several thousand milligrams of vitamin C daily for general
health.

While I respect Pauling's work, I don't recommend doses of
vitamin C greater than 1,000 milligrams a day for children, even
adolescents, except under certain special circumstances. Colds

reduce the levels of vitamin C in blood.[8] Several studies have shown that 1,000 to 2,000 milligrams a day of vitamin C can ameliorate the *severity* of colds but does not decrease the *number* of colds schoolchildren have each year.[9] Remember that 1,000 milligrams of vitamin C a day is about fifteen times the RDA, but can be readily achieved by a diet rich in fruits and vegetables; it is not a true megadose.

Vitamin C supplements in the range of 1,000 to 3,000 milligrams a day improve wound healing and general immune response in tests of immune function in humans.

Vitamin C also has a direct antiviral effect; it blocks the pathways by which viruses enter cells.

Vitamin C as a Preventive and Treatment. One thousand milligrams a day of vitamin C is a safe and reasonable (preventive) supplement for adolescents.

To *treat* severe colds, viral infections such as sore throat or bronchitis, and the flu, I find megadoses of vitamin C very effective. If your child has fever and muscle pain and is home from school, I recommend the highest dose he can take: 1,000 milligrams an hour, until he begins to get diarrhea or loose bowels. This will establish his saturation point. (Excess vitamin C causes diarrhea because it draws water into the intestines.) Stop the C until the next day, when you should give him 1,000 milligrams every two to three hours until his bowels again become loose. Stop C again until the third day, when you should give him 1,000 milligrams every four to six hours. Maintain this dose until the cold is over, then gradually cut the dose back over two weeks to 1,000 milligrams a day.

The antiviral effect of C depends on getting the highest levels possible into the tissues. *Is it safe?* Very: not only for viruses, but for acute allergic reactions as well. When should you *not* give vitamin C? If your child has kidney disease or is too sick to take food and liquid along with it.

Vitamin A and Viruses. For children over ten, vitamin A is also helpful with acute viral infections. It stimulates the immune system's killer T-cells, which kill viruses and cancer cells. The problem with vitamin A, though, is that it's *fat soluble:* it doesn't dissolve in water. For this reason, it accumulates in the body, and can become toxic. But toxicity depends on how much you take and for how long; I recommend very high doses but only for a very short time: 100,000 units a day for three to five days.

Larger or older adolescents weighing over 120 pounds can take 200,000 units a day for three to five days *maximum*.

Stop all vitamin A after three to five days. The levels in the body will slowly decrease. *Do not taper the dose off slowly; stop all at once.*

Note: I do not use this treatment with children under ten, except in special circumstances. Nor should it be used if there's a chance of pregnancy; it may contribute to birth defects. *In any case, don't use this treatment more than once every twelve weeks.*

Some children have chronic or frequent respiratory infections or sore throats. This is neither normal nor desirable. Most of these children have been overdosed with antibiotics and are suffering from allergies and yeast problems. Often there are fatty-acid and mineral deficiencies. Loren's case is typical.

Loren was a fifteen-year-old with a sore throat that had lingered for a year while she took antibiotics. Although the antibiotics had actually eliminated her original strep culture, she still had white patches on her tonsils and swollen lymph nodes in her neck that looked like signs of strep. She had lost weight and was easily fatigued. She often felt dizzy and frequently missed school.

I told her parents that the first step in Loren's recovery was to stop the antibiotics. I put Loren on a low-sugar diet, with acidophilus supplements and Nystatin to cut down on her intestinal yeast.

To restore her immune system to normal, I prescribed:

Flaxseed oil	1 Tb daily
MaxEPA (fish-oil capsules)	1,000 mg, 3 daily
Vitamin A	10,000 units daily
Vitamin C	2,000 mg daily
Magnesium chloride (Slow-Mag)	300 mg daily
Multimineral:	
Zinc	20 mg
Copper	2 mg
Selenium	100 mcg
Chromium	0 .2 mg
Manganese	10 mg

Over the next three to four months, Loren's sore throats disappeared. She gained weight and her vitality returned. This approach will help 80 to 90 percent of teenagers with chronic or recurrent respiratory or throat infections. If it doesn't work completely, an allergy evaluation should be undertaken.

MONONUCLEOSIS

Mononucleosis ("mono") is still greatly feared among teenagers. It used to be called the kissing disease, because it can be spread through saliva, but in fact it is not generally understood how most cases are transmitted. Mono is caused by the Epstein-Barr virus (EBV). EBV is possibly the most common human virus in the world. Almost everyone has been infected with it by the age of thirty-five, but most never develop clinical mononucleosis.

The classic symptoms of acute mononucleosis are severe sore throat, swollen lymph nodes (prominent in the back of the neck as well as the front), and severe fatigue with even mild exertion.

Although the throat may be full of pus, the infection is *viral*, not bacterial. Antibiotics should *not* be used; kids with acute mono are much more likely to have allergic drug reactions than kids with other infections. Rest is important; the illness may last from two weeks to several months.

The vitamin C to bowel tolerance regimen described on page 203 is very helpful in acute mono. In the convalescent phase, the following nutritional supplements are also helpful:

Magnesium	6 mg per pound per day (lower dose if diarrhea occurs)
B complex	Supplying per day: 50 mg vitamin B-6, 0.8 mg folic acid

If your child gets mono, he will be immune to it thereafter and cannot contract it again. There are some people who develop a relapse of their old infection or who go on to develop a chronic, monolike illness, the now well-known Epstein-Barr virus syndrome (CEBV). In most cases diagnosed as CEBV, the EBV is actually not the culprit, though. What's going on is obscure; the cause is either another viral infection or a more profound breakdown in immune organization. I have seen a few patients who developed acute mononucleosis in adolescence who were never quite the same afterward: their initial illness was followed by chronic fatigue, dizzy spells, intermittent fevers, sore throats, swollen glands, muscle aches, depression, anxiety, and the development of multiple allergies. Usually these patients don't seek medical attention as teenagers. They live with the symptoms and everyone thinks of them as troubled teenagers. The stress of adulthood makes them seek help.

My basic teen diet and the supplement plan for teens with chronic respiratory infections, outlined on pages 201–204, is quite helpful for many CEBV patients. *Magnesium* doses should be pushed to almost the point of diarrhea—sometimes very high doses are needed to counter the fatigue. Doses of up to 1,000 milligrams a day are safe.

B-12 injections sometimes help dramatically. They may need to be given once or twice a week, 1 milligram per dose. No toxicity has been reported with B-12, although some people feel *more* tired from it and shouldn't receive it. Positive effects are apparent within days—if they don't appear, the B-12 should be stopped immediately.

Occasionally, high doses of the B vitamin *folic acid* are helpful. The RDA for folic acid is 0.4 milligram a day, but CEBV sufferers may need up to 10 milligrams a day to feel well. *Megadoses of folic acid can be dangerous, and this treatment must be supervised by a physician who understands the risks and benefits.*

Iron deficiency is not infrequent in CEBV. Your child's doctor should check his serum ferritin level.

Viruses in the herpes family, including EBV, are nourished by an amino acid called arginine, which is found in high concentration in beans and nuts. (The cocoa bean, from which we get chocolate, is high in arginine.) But another amino acid, lysine, antagonizes arginine—prevents it from having its usual effect on a virus. For this reason, diets with a high ratio of lysine to arginine may offer some protections against recurrent herpes infections. It might make sense to have a youngster with acute mono follow such a diet until he has recovered.

High Lysine–Low Arginine Diet

Note: This is *not* a good lifetime diet. It is recommended only for a few weeks.

EAT	AVOID
Eggs	Chocolate
Cheese	Nuts
Fish	Beans
Poultry	Tofu
Meat	

CEBV can be a disabling illness, and its treatment requires professional help. It is *not common* among teenagers; if your teen is tired, there are probably other reasons for it.

FATIGUE

Fatigue is so common among teenagers, it's almost normal. If a teenager's fatigue prevents him from doing all the things he wants to, it's worthwhile making an issue out of it. The main reason teenagers get tired, in my experience, is that the nutritional demands of rapid growth and hormonal development are not met by their terrible diets. My basic diet plan has brought more than a few kids back to life.

Iron deficiency can cause fatigue long before it causes anemia, so iron should be checked out. For a menstruating girl, or for a teenager who eats little meat, it's a good idea to test for iron deficiency. A blood-ferritin test measures the level of an iron-transporting protein. Low ferritin can reveal iron deficiency before a blood count does.

Aside from iron, the most useful dietary supplements are the following:

Magnesium	3 mg per pound per day
B complex	
Vitamin B-1	15 mg
Vitamin B-6	30 mg
Folic acid	0.4 mg

To treat a tired teen whose fatigue is food-based, I recommend my basic diet plan. I would also add a magnesium supplement—3 milligrams per pound per day, and a B complex multivitamin supplying about 15 milligrams of B-1 and twice as much (30 milligrams) of B-6.

The world's oldest complaint comes in three varieties: *tension, migraine,* and *sinus.*

Tension Headaches

These originate in muscular contractions of the head and neck. They are often experienced as pressure around the forehead or top of the head that travels down the back of the neck. They may be caused by injury, poor posture, nervous tension or stress, or they may be a secondary response to migraines.

Training in muscle relaxation is very helpful in relieving tension headaches. So is a magnesium supplement. Magnesium deficiency makes tension worse in much the same way as it does menstrual cramps. I recommend magnesium in doses of up to 600 milligrams a day until the headache improves or your teenager experiences a loosening of the bowels. This is the signal that the body has reached its point of toleration. At that point, cut back the dose and continue until the headache improves.

Migraine Headaches

Caused by the constriction and dilation of blood vessels in the *covering* of the brain, they tend to come on quickly and can be very severe, lasting for several hours or days. They're often accompanied by nausea, vomiting, and an inability to tolerate bright lights. Migraines may cause secondary tension headaches, which can last for days.

Several studies have shown that *food allergy* is an important cause of migraine headaches, especially in children and teenagers.[10] Disturbances in the body's handling of *calcium,* and in the actions of *prostaglandins* are also part of the migraine syndrome, so the body's supply of calcium, magnesium,[11] and EFAs[12] have a major effect on migraine headaches.

The most dramatic migraine case I've seen was Patrick's. I saw him first when he was thirteen. He had been suffering from severe daily migraines since he was eight. He had not responded to any changes in diet or to any of a wide variety of drugs he had been given. At times, the constant pain made him so depressed that he considered suicide.

Patrick had some other problems as well. He hadn't grown significantly in three years, nor had he yet reached puberty. His doctor consulted me because of some very strange blood test results: The fatty acid levels in Patrick's serum and red blood cells were totally out of balance with each other.

My diagnosis was that Patrick would require very large doses of omega-3 EFAs in the form of fish-oil capsules. I recommended 16 grams a day of MaxEPA capsules.

The result was remarkable: over the next few months, Patrick's headaches began to subside. As they did, we gradually lowered his dosage of MaxEPA capsules to 5 grams a day. To everyone's amazement, within three months after treatment began, Patrick also began to grow and develop sexually. Within a year, he had caught up with his peers.

A year later, I read a report from the University of Indiana on the use of high doses of fish oils to treat migraine headaches. Patrick's case, obviously, was far from unique.

Note: I would not recommend very high doses of fish oils without medical supervision. But you can safely give any teen with chronic migraine headaches nutritional doses of MaxEPA (about 3 grams a day) or flaxseed oil (1 tablespoon a day), as well as magnesium (3 milligrams a day per pound of body weight). If your teenager doesn't respond, then you should investigate the possibility of a food allergy.

Sinus Headaches

Sinus headaches are almost always allergic in origin. The pain is concentrated around the eyes and in the cheeks; it may also travel to the back of the head. Sinus headaches are often associated with nasal congestion or postnasal drip, and tend to be worse in damp weather. They may improve somewhat with decongestants or antihistamines.

Chronic sinus headaches are usually caused by allergy to molds in the air or to foods, or both. Airborne molds are concentrated in damp places such as basements, swamps, and forests. They're also more prevalent during early spring and fall, especially when the humidity is high. Mold counts go up dramatically just before a storm.

Mold allergy usually requires treatment by a good allergist, but you can help relieve your teen's sinus headaches by eliminating foods containing molds and the molds' close cousin, yeast.

- *Sugar* feeds yeast; your teenager should not only avoid table sugar and sweets, but also natural sugars found in fruits, fruit juices, milk, and products made from flour, such as bread and crackers.
- *Bread, cheese, prepared foods* such as soups that contain yeast or yeast extract, and *vitamins* made from yeast.
- *Fermented foods.* Yeast activates fermentation to produce alcohol and vinegar. Hidden sources of alcohol include cough syrups and vanilla extract. Vinegar is found in commercial sauces, catsup, mayonnaise, salad dressings, soy sauce, and in sauerkraut and other pickled vegetables. Read all product labels for ingredients.
- *Naturally occurring yeast* and *mold* abound on the skins of some fruits, vegetables, seeds, peanuts, and so on. Avoid dried fruit and commercial fruit juices—apple cider is so yeasty that, untreated, it will ferment in a day or two at room temperature. Peel all root vegetables and remove the outer leaves of lettuce and cabbage. Nut butters are okay, but watch out for peanuts (especially prone to the cancer-causing mold aflatoxin) and other shelled nuts.

What's allowed then? Meat, fish, poultry, eggs, all fresh vegetables (except mushrooms), rice, potatoes, oats, rice cakes, nut butters.

You can decrease the growth of yeast in the intestine with any of the following natural substances:

- *Acidophilus.* I recommend freeze-dried Primedophilus from Klaire Laboratories, available in health-food stores. Take ½ teaspoon a day before eating.
- *Caprylic acid.* I recommend Capricin in 300-milligram capsules, from Probiologic, available in health-food stores. Since it may be a bit irritating to the intestine, I recommend it be taken with food. Start your teenager with one pill twice a day at breakfast and dinner. Increase by one pill every day up to a dose of twelve pills a day—six at breakfast, six at dinner. After

two months at twelve pills a day, slowly decrease the dose to zero.

- *Garlic oil.* Do *not* use deodorized garlic oil. A good choice is Arizona Natural Garlic capsules, which are rich in the yeast-killing compound allicin. Take nine to twelve capsules a day. Sometimes, when this treatment is started, the allergic symptoms worsen for a few days and then start to improve.

As soon as your teenager's symptoms start to clear up on any of the above, you can gradually reintroduce—one at a time—to your teenager's diet the foods that have been removed: nuts, seeds, fresh fruit, milk. Then begin to introduce vinegar, bread, and cheese. Continue to avoid only those foods that bring on the headaches.

If the symptoms don't improve after two weeks with this treatment, you may need to consult a doctor who understands yeast allergy.

Bonus: This treatment may also aid migraine sufferers.

Prevent Yeast Problems Before They Start. Be careful about exposing your youngster to antibiotics and sugar. If for some reason antibiotics are necessary, follow the treatment with two weeks of:

Acidophilus: ½ teaspoon Primedophilus twice daily
Caprylic acid: six Capricin pills with breakfast and supper (twelve a day)
Garlic oil: three capsules of Arizona Natural Garlic with each meal
Or have your doctor prescribe *oral Nystatin.*

IRRITABLE BOWEL SYNDROME

Irritable bowel syndrome, which produces abdominal pain, bloating, constipation, diarrhea, and, sometimes, mucus in the stool, is usually attributed to anxiety. It is the commonest intestinal disorder in the United States, and usually begins in adolescence. It can certainly produce an irritable teenager, and severe cases can be disabling. My experience is that anxiety generally does play a small but definite role, depending on how severe the stress is. Some other factors are always worth searching for.

Abnormal Intestinal Flora or Fauna

Common to two-thirds of irritable bowel syndrome cases is an abnormal level of intestinal flora or fauna, including a lack of healthy bacteria and an overgrowth of yeast or the presence of parasites. Treatment can produce dramatic relief.

Some Questions to Ask: Has the teenager been treated with antibiotics, which, you will recall, can lead to a yeast overgrowth? Are there signs of yeast overgrowth, such as a rash around the anus or, in a girl, a vaginal discharge?

Has the teenager traveled to places such as Mexico where he could pick up parasites? Has he gone camping in the mountains? Clear, beautiful mountain streams are often contaminated with the common parasite *Giardia lamblia.* Children are especially prone to intestinal infection by this parasite, which causes a mucus diarrhea, abdominal pain, and weight loss in its acute stages but may cause constipation and gassiness in the chronic phase.

It's not easy to diagnose intestinal parasites, because stool samples are often misleading. The most reliable method I've found is the Bueno-Parrish Method, published in the *American Journal of Proctocology, Gastroenterology and Colon and Rectal Surgery* in 1981. If you suspect parasites in your teenager, refer your physician to it.[13] This examination can now be performed through Medical Diagnostic Laboratory, 3544 Conner Street, Bronx, N.Y. 10461.

Food Allergy or Food Intolerance

These are present in almost all cases, but the standard diets don't take this into account.[14] The major offenders are dairy products, glutenous grains such as wheat, oats, barley, and rye; and yeast- and mold-containing foods. Also important are fruits, nuts, and beans.

By far the most common allergy is to *milk.* There are two kinds of milk intolerance: *lactose intolerance* and *milk-protein allergy.* Lactose (milk sugar) intolerance is created when there aren't enough enzymes in the intestine to break down milk sugar (lactose). Instead, intestinal bacteria break it down, making lactic acid that irritates the intestine, producing abdominal pain, gas, and diarrhea. Lactose intolerance may be inherited, or it may develop when some other illness, such as an infection, destroys the enzymes that break down lactose.

Since there is more lactose in whole milk or cream than in hard cheese, young people with lactose intolerance may be able to tolerate cheese.

Milk-protein intolerance is an allergic reaction to one of the proteins found in milk, and may show up also as a severe intolerance to cheese. Symptoms range from itching, wheezing, and headache to abdominal pain, gas, and constipation or diarrhea. Lactose intolerance, by making the intestine more porous, may itself cause milk-protein allergy and possibly other food allergies as well.[15]

Questions to Ask: Is the teenager allergic? Does he or she have hay fever or asthma, a postnasal drip, skin rashes, or itching?

Overproduction of Prostaglandins and Calcium-Generated Spasms

These spasms have nothing to do with how much calcium your teen consumes; they are caused by magnesium deficiency. Prostaglandin overproduction, of course, is an imbalance caused by an EFA deficiency. I often find deficiencies of omega-3 EFAs and magnesium in teens with irritable bowel syndrome. Together, they contribute to the severity of the symptoms.

Questions to Ask: Are there signs of an essential fatty acid deficiency, such as dry or rough skin, brittle nails, or menstrual cramps? Are there signs of magnesium deficiency, such as muscle spasms and / or twitches?

Wade is a good illustration of how to track down the many causes of irritable bowel syndrome. For three years, ever since an acute illness diagnosed as food poisoning, this fourteen-year-old had suffered from chronic diarrhea and abdominal pain. Wade's doctor had treated the food poisoning with an antibiotic, and although Wade's fever had subsided, the accompanying diarrhea became worse.

When Wade tested positive on a lactose tolerance test, his doctor put him on a low-lactose, milk-free diet, but he didn't really improve. Although he took large quantities of antidiarrheal and antispasmodic drugs every day, he could not lick his symptoms.

I learned that Wade had done a lot of skiing in the Rockies and that as an infant he had frequently been given antibiotics for ear infections. As a child he had suffered from hay fever and mild asthma, but had outgrown his asthma.

I started Wade on a milk gluten– and yeast– and mold–elimination diet. This reduced his symptoms by 70 percent, allowing a 50 percent reduction of medication. But we found that if he deviated from the diet at all, he would come down with severe abdominal pain.

We added acidophilus and Capricin. Wade reported three bad days, and then began to improve somewhat. He was able to stop his medication completely.

When we added flaxseed oil and magnesium, no immediate change was apparent, although Wade's hair became less dry.

A parasite exam revealed cysts of *Giardia lamblia* parasite, which is common in the Colorado mountains. We treated this condition with the drug Atabrine for seven days.

Now Wade's food tolerance began to improve; he was able to eat fruits, nuts, and grains. Milk, however, remained a problem. A skin test showed that Wade was allergic to milk protein, so we began a series of desensitizing injections.

Wade was by now virtually problem free. As a bonus, the following spring his hay fever was better than it had ever been.

Wade's story shows how complex the causes of irritable bowel syndrome can be. Here we had a young teenager who, as a child, had had allergies and had been deficient in omega-3 EFAs. His allergies led to recurrent ear infections, which were treated with antibiotics. The antibiotics, in turn, produced a yeast overgrowth that led to a yeast allergy that manifested itself in mild asthma and worse hay fever. To cap all this, Wade picked up a *Giardia lamblia* infection that produced acute gastroenteritis, which left him with a lactose intolerance. The *Giardia lamblia* was misdiagnosed as food poisoning and treated with antibiotics, which brought back the yeast overgrowth.

Wade's intestines were now inflamed; the yeast overgrowth added to the inflammation and activated the *Giardia* infection.

(It's known that *Candida*, the intestinal yeast, stimulates *Giardia* growth.)

With this series of events, intestinal function breakdown was inevitable, and with it, new food allergies developed.

What was the cause of Wade's irritable bowel syndrome? Pick something—anything—from the list above, and you'll be right on track.

Fatigue, headache, and irritable bowel syndrome often occur together. Consequently, their nutritional roots are often the same. They can be associated with anxiety, depression, and emotional stress. If you're concerned about them, read the next section very carefully.

BEHAVIORAL AND ACADEMIC PROBLEMS

The various pressures on your teen—hormonal, social, academic, athletic—can produce reactions ranging from problems in concentrating on schoolwork to confusion, anxiety, depression, and aggression. Usually, such problems are temporary, but if they persist, it's time for concern. If your teenager's schoolwork deteriorates, if he has trouble sleeping at night or suddenly loses weight, if he starts to withdraw from friends and school activities, if he becomes involved in drug or alcohol abuse or gets into scrapes with the police, if he is fatigued or has headaches or abdominal pain as well, you will need to take action.

Many of these problems have underlying nutritional causes, but before we explore those, you will need to ask yourself whether you are giving your child plenty of nurturing attention. Adolescents need that if they are to give their best in school, in their social lives, or on the athletic field.

Now that most parents work, time for children must often be consciously scheduled, as it may need to be if you have more than one child. Give each child just a few minutes of undivided attention each day—that's usually all a teenager needs.

The Nutrition Connection

There is no question that nutrition can be an important factor in a broad range of behavioral problems. Sociologist Stephen Schoenthaler has demonstrated that dietary changes as simple, in many cases, as replacing soda with orange juice, can significantly decrease aggressive behavior among boys held in juvenile detention centers.[16]

In most cases, I would expect my basic low-fat, low-sugar, high-fiber diet plan, with flaxseed oil (or cod-liver or walnut oil) and magnesium supplements, to help teenagers with concentration, depression, or poor impulse control. The brain has a high concentration of omega-3 EFAs; they are important for the normal activity of nerve tissue.

But sometimes a broader program of nutritional supplementation is necessary. Two key elements are B vitamins and amino acids.

The brain uses B vitamins for building neurotransmitters and for providing energy. A combination that can significantly affect concentration, memory, and mood in some teens consists of

B VITAMINS

B-1	25 mg daily
B-6	50 mg daily
Folic acid	0.4 mg daily
B-12	1 mg daily in sublingual tablets that dissolve under the tongue

Amino acids are the building blocks of protein. In the body, proteins are used to make everything from cell receptors to the neurotransmitters that carry messages from brain cell to brain cell. Most American youngsters consume a lot of protein, so that we don't usually have to worry about amino acid deficiencies. But when I studied a number of emotionally troubled adolescents who were eating high-protein diets, I found that, contrary to expectation, many of them were excreting very small quantities of amino acids in their urine.

I suspect that in such cases, one or more food allergies are interfering with the proper digestion of protein, and that means that the formation of vital neurotransmitters may be impaired. Since our thoughts and feelings travel over neural circuits, anything that impairs neurotransmitter formation is going to affect deeply how we think and feel, as well as how we behave.

Taking amino acids as supplements may have a noticeable effect on levels of neurotransmitters in the brain, and so can help relieve symptoms ranging from difficulty in concentration to depression and other behavioral problems.

A variety of supplements can affect memory and concentration:

- *Choline.* This amino acid is used by the brain to make acetylcholine, the key neurotransmitter involved in memory. Choline supplements improve memory in humans and animals. Choline is normally found in such foods as liver, eggs, oatmeal, tofu, lentils, and split peas.

   Supplements of 1,000 milligrams a day are totally safe, except during pregnancy. Choline may be taken as plain choline capsules or as lecithin capsules, phosphatidylcholine. A good dose of phosphatidylcholine is 1,000 milligrams three or more times a day. (Lecithin capsules are less than one-third choline.)

- *Pantothenic acid.* The body also uses this B vitamin to make acetylcholine. Pantothenic acid is found in liver, kidneys, oatmeal, brown rice, lentils, tofu, broccoli, mushrooms, avocado, cabbage, peas, cauliflower, trout, and dark-meat turkey.

   High doses of pantothenic acid improve wound healing and work with choline to enhance mental concentration. There are *no* side effects. Doses of 500 milligrams two to three times a day are always well tolerated.

- *Glutamine.* This is an amino acid that enters the brain rapidly and is used as fuel. It is also converted to glutamic acid, an amino acid that stimulates the brain's response to acetylcholine. Glutamine should not be given to children with seizure disorders or liver disease; otherwise it is very safe. The dose is about 250 milligrams a day.

Depression. Don't try to treat a depressed teenager by yourself. *Professional guidance is essential.* Four amino acids, used by the brain in making neurotransmitters, may be helpful in the nutritional treatment of depression: tryptophan, tyrosine, phenylalanine, and methionine. But their use is quite tricky—they should be given *only* under the guidance of a psychologist or physician familiar with their vagaries.

The Allergy Connection

If you've read this book through, it won't surprise you to read that allergies to foods, molds, and yeast can play major roles in creating and sustaining behavioral problems in adolescents.[17]

If your child has difficulty concentrating in school and does not respond to a regimen of amino acids and pantothenic acid, suspect allergy, especially to foods or molds, and provide some therapy accordingly. (See above, pp. 209–10 under Headaches.)

More serious behavior problems in teenagers can also be linked to food allergy, yeast infection, poor diet, and nutritional deficiencies. In such cases, a stable, supportive family can be crucial to the success of nutritional therapy. Unfortunately, such was not the case with Terry.

When I first met Terry, she was a confused fifteen-year-old whose parents were divorced. Her mother had become a prostitute, and Terry lived with her father and stepmother.

Essentially, Terry had a bad self-image. Because she wanted to be liked, she was easily influenced by her peers. She smoked heavily and drank lots of coffee. She also ate a nutritionally deficient diet.

In my office, she showed signs of immaturity. She giggled a great deal and could not sit still. She was doing very poorly in school and was subject to mood swings, including depression and irritability. To add to her problems, she had acne, although fortunately it was a mild case.

Over the years Terry had been given a lot of antibiotics for strep throats, bronchitis, and hay fever. Her blood tests showed a vitamin B-6 deficiency.

I had many threads to weave with Terry. I got her to agree to drink less coffee, eat fewer sweets, and take the nutritional supplements I find helpful with distressed adolescents:

B complex supplying 50 mg per day of vitamin B-6

Vitamin E	400 units
Vitamin C	1,000 mg
Magnesium	400 mg
Zinc	20 mg
Copper	1 mg
Manganese	10 mg
Selenium	100 mcg
Chromium	400 mcg
Flaxseed oil	1 Tb (or 1 teaspoon cod-liver oil or 2 Tb walnut oil)

Terry's father reported that she was far less twitchy on these supplements, but I didn't notice any significant change in behavior on her next office visit. Because of her long history of antibiotic use and because her skin tests showed allergies to several yeasts and molds, I recommended that she go on a yeast-free diet and that she use the yeast-killing drug Nystatin.

Terry had a remarkable response to Nystatin. During her next visit she no longer giggled, and she could sit still! There was also a significant change in her behavior at home and in school.

Sadly, though, after a few weeks Terry stopped taking the Nystatin. She found a new boyfriend and started smoking and drinking coffee again, and this led to a relapse. Soon after, she ran away from home.

When she was found and brought back, her father had her committed to a psychiatric hospital. I discussed her case with the attending psychiatrists and they agreed to test Nystatin's effects on her. First they began a month of observation to get a baseline analysis of her negative and self-destructive behavior. Then they restarted her on the Nystatin and reported that they had observed measurable improvements in her behavior.

You may have noticed that I treated Terry's behavior problem in almost exactly the same way as Loren's sore throat. That was no accident; it underlies the most important message in this book. As said on page 1, children have a remarkable ability to heal themselves; doctors and medications do not make them better. When a child is given penicillin for a strep throat, it is not penicillin that cures the infection, it is the child's immune system. The penicillin may make it a bit easier, but controlled studies have failed to show that the child gets better much faster with penicillin than without it. Similarly, nutrition does not cure disease. Optimum nutrition merely allows a child to heal himself as effectively as possible.

Most chronic illness, from chronic sore throat to headache and anxiety, results from a child's inability to heal himself. In our culture there are a number of stumbling blocks to effective self-healing. Some of these are so common that they affect most sick children: dietary deficiencies of omega-3 EFAs and magnesium, plus excessive consumption of sugar, refined carbohydrates, and processed fats and oils. Various mineral deficiencies (iron, copper, zinc, selenium) are close behind.

Excessive use of antibiotics is another huge barrier to self-healing; it causes a loss of normal bacteria and an overgrowth of undesirable microorganisms, especially yeast. Yeast overgrowth can lead to yeast allergy.

Correcting EFA or mineral deficiencies or yeast over-growth problems does not cure disease; it allows your child to heal himself by removing the impediments that were making him sick. It doesn't matter what the particular illness is—*we're not treating the illness, we're treating the child.* If you understand this principle, the next chapter should come as no surprise. The same nutritional aids that allow your child to bounce back from childhood illness also help to prevent the common degenerative diseases of adulthood.

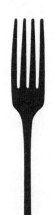

How Power-Packed Nutrition Creates Immunity for Life

9

Health is more than the absence of disease. Health is the vitality that confers resistance to chronic disease. Nowhere is this easier to see than in the face of a happy child at play. Her vitality is nourished by lots of love and imaginative play; optimum nutrition will help her to maintain it into adulthood. A wonderful dividend of the nutrition plan in this book is that, in addition to helping you raise a disease-resistant child, it will help your child avoid the most common and dangerous degenerative diseases of adulthood.

Each age has its characteristic diseases. In childhood, infection and allergy are the commonest; they represent a malfunction of the immune system. In allergy, some immune responses are abnormally hyperactive, whereas in chronic infection, other immune responses are not active enough. It is important to understand that these two conditions often occur together. The problem is not usually that the immune system as a whole is too strong or too weak, rather, it is *disorganized*.

Immune disorganization contributes to some of the commonest and most lethal adult diseases. On one side, there are the diseases of inflammation: arthritis, colitis, multiple sclerosis, and

221

autoimmune diseases such as lupus. Sadly, all these disorders, in which the body's immune system turns against the body's own organs, are increasing among young adults at an alarming rate.

On the other side lies cancer, until AIDS the most feared disease of this century. In cancer, the immune system fails to destroy defective cells that form continuously in the body. Normally, patrolling white blood cells zap them before they gain a foothold; when the immune response fails, the defective cells grow unchecked.

It is worth noting that people with cancer are more likely to develop autoimmune disease, and vice versa. As diseases of immune disorganization, cancer and inflammatory diseases are the degenerative adult counterparts of chronic infection and allergy. Throughout life, there is no environmental factor more important to a well-regulated immune system than a diet that properly balances EFAs and the co-factor nutrients that govern their metabolism.

The largest group of adult diseases are those that primarily affect circulation: arteriosclerosis, hypertension, and diabetes. All these conditions damage the body by decreasing blood flow to vital organs. Fatty deposits, thickened linings, and overgrowths of fibrous tissue all narrow blood vessels in the heart, kidneys, and brain. In diabetes, the major factor in circulatory damage is an excessive level of sugar in the blood; in hypertension, it is high blood pressure. In arteriosclerosis, the major factors are still controversial, but high blood levels of cholesterol and chronic psychological stress play important roles.

None of these disorders is primarily caused by impaired immune function, but they all involve the same derangements in cell chemistry that cause immune-system disorganization. If you look at the individual cells involved and at the prostaglandins they make—which, in turn, govern their growth and functioning— amazing similarities emerge among allergy, cancer, and circulatory disease. The scientific evidence suggests that all of today's common diseases are caused by a common set of biochemical disturbances that have reached epidemic proportions in our culture. These disturbances produce different diseases in different people, depending on their inherited predisposition, their life experiences, and the quality of their nutrition.

Chronic degenerative diseases don't just happen; they develop invisibly over the course of many, many years. In addition to helping you make sure you have the healthiest possible child, the nutritional guidelines I've given you in this book are designed to safeguard her from chronic degenerative disease as she matures. In this chapter, I will look specifically at these three groups of diseases and pinpoint the scientific evidence that shows how my diet of high-fiber, low-sugar, low-fat, EFA-and-mineral-rich foods can protect against chronic disease in adulthood.

DISEASES OF INFLAMMATION AND AUTOIMMUNITY

A great deal of my clinical practice is involved with patients suffering from autoimmune diseases or chronic inflammatory conditions whose causes are as yet unknown to science. I've found that very often these conditions are accompanied by unsuspected nutritional deficiencies. In fact, it was through my work with such patients that I learned firsthand how important nutrition is to the practice of medicine. Working with these patients was the initial stimulus to do research on the therapeutic role of EFAs, magnesium, and the antioxidant nutrients. Clinical studies by other researchers, epidemiologic studies, and animal experiments have all confirmed my observations. (Epidemiologists investigate the distribution of diseases in different populations.)

EFAs. Fat is an issue in most inflammatory diseases. Multiple sclerosis, for example, is associated with diets high in saturated fats.[1] In British studies, patients with multiple sclerosis[2] and rheumatoid arthritis[3] have consistently improved when saturated fats were removed from their diets. When essential fatty acids were *added* to their diets, they improved even more.[4] Several studies have now shown that omega-3 EFAs, in the form of Max-EPA fish-oil extract capsules, work especially well for arthritic patients.[5]

A study reported two years ago in the *New England Journal of Medicine*[6] seems to explain why. EFAs, you will recall, are metabolized by the body into prostaglandins, the chemicals that regulate virtually every system in our bodies, including our immune systems. The omega-3 EFAs in fish oils, it turns out, block the formation of the particular prostaglandins that create inflammation.

In multiple sclerosis, on the other hand, plant-based EFAs, such as the omega-6s in safflower, black currant, and primrose oils, can alleviate some of the symptoms and their underlying biochemical abnormalities.[7]

While these clinical studies don't prove that EFAs can actually *prevent* immune diseases, some epidemiologic and experimental data suggest that they can. Autoimmune and inflammatory diseases are rare among populations whose diets are high in EFAs and low in saturated fats—as is the traditional Japanese diet. At the same time, the incidence of these diseases is increasing in industrialized nations whose citizens eat a lot of saturated fats and few omega-3s. In animal experiments, mice and rats bred to develop autoimmune diseases were fed diets rich in fish oils. The results? They either didn't get the diseases they were genetically programmed to develop, or they got very mild cases.[8]

Selenium. While data on other nutrients is skimpy, some interesting Danish studies have shown that people with rheumatoid arthritis have low levels of selenium in their blood. Given selenium in supplements, some patients improve.[9]

ARTERIOSCLEROSIS, HYPERTENSION, AND DIABETES

All three of these diseases radically affect the circulatory system—they cause heart attacks and heart failure, kidney damage, and strokes. Their nutritional antecedents have been extensively researched and, once again, fat is a crucial issue.

EFAs. Almost everyone knows by now that arteriosclerosis is associated with high levels of cholesterol in the blood. Many people, though, are not aware that the culprit is not so much the cholesterol in food as it is the saturated fats. High cholesterol levels in the blood, arteriosclerosis, and hypertension have all been *independently* linked to a diet high in nonessential saturated fats. Omega-3 EFAs, such as those found in fatty deep-water fish such as salmon and tuna and in MaxEPA fish-oil extract capsules, lower cholesterol and triglyceride levels and blood pressure. What's more, they actually protect against the development of both hypertension and arteriosclerosis. Omega-6 EFAs, found in vegetable oils such as safflower, black currant, or evening primrose oil, have a similar effect.[10]

How do EFAs achieve this magical result? By actually alter-ing the chemistry of the body. Once again, it's a question of prostaglandins. Saturated animal fats found in red meat, poultry skin, butter, and cream, or saturated vegetable fats found in palm or coconut oil, or *any* oil that, although it might have been origi-nally unsaturated, has been wholly or partially hydrogenated, spur the production of prostaglandins, which makes blood thicker and more easily coagulated and constricts blood vessels. EFAs, both omega-3 and omega-6, have *exactly the opposite effect;* they trigger production of the prostaglandins that *enlarge* blood ves-sels and make the blood less sticky. A diet high in saturated fats is guaranteed to set up conditions that are just right for the development of arteriosclerosis and hypertension. Replacing these fats with EFAs does just the opposite.

Salt. Both epidemiological studies and laboratory experi-ments offer abundant proof that animals and people who consume a lot of sodium chloride, or common table salt, are far more likely to have high blood pressure than those who don't. Since sodium chloride is universally added to manufactured foods in large quan-tities, it's crucial to read labels carefully before using any food in a can, bottle, or package.

Magnesium and the Fatty-Acid Connection. Magnesium is a key mineral in the prevention of high blood pressure. Drs. Bur-ton and Bella Altura of New York's Downstate Medical Center have shown that animals fed a magnesium-deficient diet develop high blood pressure. The Alturas believe that magnesium defi-ciency lies behind much human hypertension as well. The catch is that once you've got hypertension, magnesium alone won't do much good, because the changes in blood vessels are irreversible.

Magnesium can't protect you against high blood pressure if you eat a lot of saturated fat, either. Mildred Seelig, executive director of the American College of Nutrition, has observed that saturated fat actually blocks the absorption of magnesium from the intestines. But—you guessed it—EFAs *increase* the amount of magnesium you absorb from food or supplements.

Many studies support Seelig's observation. Animal studies, especially those of Dr. Yves Rayssiguier in France, have found that magnesium deficiency raises the levels of cholesterol and total fat in the blood.[11] Studies of humans have shown that magnesium supplements raise the level of the "good" cholesterol, high-density lipoprotein, or HDL, that protects against heart disease. What's more, magnesium deficiency can be found in the majority of patients with heart disease, diabetes, and high blood pressure. It's not known whether the deficiency causes the disease or is caused by it.[12] The causes of heart and blood-vessel disease are complex, but it does appear that *a diet low in sodium chloride and high in magnesium and potassium will prevent hypertension and vascular diseases, especially if it is also rich in EFAs and low in nonessential fats.* These are all characteristics of my basic diet plan.

Fiber. Soluble fibers, such as those found in oats, beans, vegetables (such as cabbage), and fruits (such as apples), tend to lower both cholesterol and blood sugar. For this reason, Dr. John Anderson of the University of Kentucky Medical Center has pioneered the use of low-fat, high-fiber, high-carbohydrate diets for diabetics. Fats can worsen such complications of diabetes as high blood pressure and arteriosclerosis, and Anderson was dismayed at the amount of fat in the American Diabetic Association's recommended diet. His group has found that in addition to lowering blood-sugar levels in diabetics, his diets lower fat and cholesterol levels in diabetics and nondiabetics alike. They also stabilize blood sugar in people prone to hypoglycemia, a pathological drop in blood sugar that produces weakness, confusion, and unconsciousness.

Soluble fiber achieves its effects partly because, unlike many nutrients, it is not absorbed through the walls of the intestine. Instead, bacteria metabolize it and transform it into short-chain fatty acids. These are absorbed through the wall of the large intestine and enter the blood, which carries them to the liver, the organ that makes cholesterol and blood fat. The short-chain fatty acids signal the liver to stop producing cholesterol and other fats.

In addition, fiber-rich complex carbohydrates take longer to digest than high-sugar, simple starches such as candy or cake. That means that high-fiber carbohydrates release sugar into the blood at a slow, sustained rate rather than all at once.

When Emanuel Cheraskin was teaching at the University of Alabama School of Dentistry, he measured his colleagues' blood-sugar levels several times a day for a month. When the dentists followed their usual diets, their blood-sugar levels fluctuated wildly throughout the day even though none of them was diabetic. But when they switched to a low-sugar, high-fiber diet, their blood-sugar levels stabilized.

Some scientists speculate that a low-sugar, high-fiber diet will actually help prevent diabetes and arteriosclerosis even in people who are genetically susceptible to these killer diseases. Epidemiologic evidence bears this out.[13] Why? Because a stable blood-sugar level requires less insulin. When blood-sugar levels rise, the pancreas releases insulin into the blood, which drives the sugar out of the blood and into the cells, which use it for energy. Over time, repeated sugar zaps can exhaust a weak pancreas. In diabetes mellitus, the pancreas can't make enough insulin to keep blood-sugar levels down.

Insulin also stimulates liver and fat cells to make more fat. So when you eat a lot of sugar, you might as well be eating fat, too. A low-sugar, high-fiber diet avoids all these pitfalls.

Not all the epidemiological and experimental evidence supports the theory that fiber can prevent diabetes and atherosclerosis. But if diabetes can be treated with a diet that is typical of entire populations who seldom develop it, it seems reasonable that following such a diet from an early age could prevent some susceptible individuals from developing the disease.

Vitamin B-6. This is an important co-factor nutrient, enabling the body to metabolize EFAs into prostaglandins. Because it gums up EFA metabolism, B-6 deficiency also worsens the effects of EFA deficiencies. Vitamin B-6 deficiency in experimental animals speeds the rate at which they develop arteriosclerosis. In addition, animals with vitamin B-6 deficiency have high levels of a toxic amino acid, homocysteine, in their blood. In humans, high blood levels of this amino acid are associated with the development of severe arteriosclerosis at an early age.

Whole grains are the best food source of B-6. Many people will need to take B-6 supplements to get the full amount they need, 10 milligrams or more a day, five or more times the RDA.

Selenium. Heart-disease patients have lower levels of selenium in their blood than do healthy controls.[14] Depletion of selenium from the soil of much farmland in the United States has decreased the selenium content of grains, so that the American diet is marginally deficient. You can get the selenium you need, about 150 micrograms a day, from fish; if you don't like fish you may need a supplement.

Copper. Most Americans consume less copper than the 1 to 2 milligrams daily RDA. On the other hand, varying amounts of copper are found in drinking water, leached in from copper pipes.

Copper deficiency elevates cholesterol levels and weakens the walls of arteries. Experimental copper deprivation leads to abnormal EFA metabolism. A recent unpublished study of copper depletion in healthy young men was stopped when several of them developed heart problems.

CANCER

Cancer represents a failure of the immune system. Our bodies continuously produce small numbers of cancer cells, but usually our white blood cells promptly destroy them. When the immune system is disorganized, a person's susceptibility to cancer is increased.

Major cancers in the United States are breast, colon, uterine, prostate, and lung. With the exception of lung cancer, which is caused almost entirely by cigarette smoking and is rare in non-smokers, all of these major killers are largely influenced by diet. (Even lung cancer is to some extent affected by diet.) The following guidelines are aimed at helping you reduce your child's risk of developing cancer at any time in her life.

Fat. As a step toward reducing the frequency of colon, prostate, breast, uterine, and ovarian cancers, the National Research Council of the National Academy of Sciences recommended in 1982 that Americans cut their fat consumption by 25 percent. These recommendations were based on the results of both animal experiments and epidemiological studies. The latter consistently show that breast, colon, and reproductive-tract cancers occur more frequently in population groups that eat high-fat diets than in those that don't.[15] Epidemiology alone can't establish cause and effect, because high-fat diets are also associated with many other factors that may contribute to cancer—pollution, stress, and a decrease in breast-feeding among women. All these factors are consequences of industrialization. Hundreds of animal experiments in which rats fed both high- and low-fat diets are exposed to *carcinogenic* (cancer-promoting) substances have also shown that *the more fat in the diet, the greater the risk of cancer.* What's more, a high-fat diet produces more and bigger tumors.

As we've seen, though, not all fats are equal—there are good as well as bad fats. The exceptions, of course, are the polyunsaturated omega-3 EFAs. These essential fatty acids have to come from food; the body can't make them. This, in fact, is why they are essential. One particular omega-3 EFA, eicosapentaenoic acid (EPA), is found in the oil of such cold-water fish as mackerel, salmon, and sardines, who derive it from the plankton on which they feed.

A number of epidemiological studies have shown that when people consume a lot of EPA, they have low rates of breast cancer. This is true of Eskimos who still eat the traditional diet, high in oily northern fish that are loaded with omega-3 EFA-rich fat. Experiments have shown that omega-3 EFAs can protect against breast and colonic cancers in animals.[16]

Fiber. Tribal black South Africans who eat a traditional diet high in roots and vegetables rarely get colon cancer. But as they move to the cities they change their diets, eating less fiber and more fat and sugar. The more closely their diet matches that of white South Africans, the higher their rate of colon cancer. Exactly the same is true of black and Puerto Rican populations in this country.[17] In animal experiments, rats fed tumor-promoting chemicals developed fewer colon cancers when bran was added to their diets. The protective ingredient here is insoluble fiber of the kind found in whole wheat and crunchy vegetables.

Seed Foods. These are the seeds of plants, such as rice, corn, and beans. Dr. Walter Troll, professor of environmental medicine at New York University School of Medicine, has described a low rate of colon, breast, and prostate cancer in populations consuming large amounts of such foods. He thinks that enzymes contained in seeds inhibit tumor development.

Other compounds in seed foods, called lectins, may also protect against cancer by stimulating immune response in the intestinal tract. They probably do this by triggering the multiplication of such lymphocytes as killer and helper T-cells, which can kill tumors themselves or direct the production of antibodies against them. (For more on T-cells and the workings of the immune system, see Chapter 1.)

One Dutch study found that death from cancer in general—not just colon cancer—was *three times higher* in men on a low-fiber diet than in those who ate a lot of fiber.[18] This study was carefully controlled to make sure that the effect could not be related to any other factor, such as high or low fat intake.

The Antioxidants: Vitamins A, C, and E; Selenium. As you will recall from Chapter 1, the antioxidant defense system helps protect lymphocytes from incinerating themselves when they burn off toxins and other invaders we eat or breathe in. It also quenches the "sparks," or free radicals, that are given off when lymphocytes do their work and that, unchecked, can damage chromosomes, enzymes, and cell membranes. A great deal of experimental evidence suggests that the damage free radicals do can contribute to the development of cancer.

Epidemiological studies show that people who develop cancer in general, especially of the lung or esophagus, consume fewer of these vital antioxidants and have lower levels of them in their blood. Other studies show that, in rats, antioxidants can actively prevent the development of several common kinds of tumors. When the antioxidants are withdrawn from their diets, the rats get more and bigger tumors.[19]

This chapter has had one very simple purpose: to assure you that the nutritional recommendations in this book have a double benefit. My diet guidelines were designed to help you raise children in the best possible health and with the strongest possible immune systems. As a very substantial dividend, this program will also help protect your children against the major killer and degenerative diseases that wait to strike adults. Optimal nutrition in childhood is a gift that lasts a lifetime.

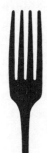

Recipes—
Including Snacks, Desserts, and Spreads:
Your Greatest Challenge

There are dozens of cookbooks devoted to healthful, natural cooking. The purpose of this chapter is not to supplant them, but to establish some basic principles and to provide recipes for the standard meal plans. The recipes presented here are all you need to get started, but are in no way limiting. Your imagination and creativity can guide you well if you have a sound understanding of the principles explained below. I emphasize snacks, desserts, and spreads because they present your greatest challenge.

BASIC INFORMATION

BREAKFASTS

Dinner would make the best breakfast for an active, growing child. Custom limits breakfast foods, however. Various cereals, breads and rolls, fruit, milk, eggs, and smoked meats (sausage and bacon) are accepted as breakfast foods. While eggs are a good source of protein, vitamin A, iron, and zinc, they are low in fiber and magnesium, and too high in cholesterol to be eaten daily. Served with whole-grain flours in pancakes and waffles or with whole-grain breads, they are fine up to twice a week. (Toddlers may eat them more frequently.)

The rest of the meals will usually be built around cereals, and if whole grains—rich in fiber, protein, and B vitamins—are used, the trick is to enhance their protein and mineral content with either milk products or seeds and nuts. So there are several recipes that present cereal-based high-protein breakfast foods.

SUPPERS

These are usually the easiest. A hot meal combining a high-protein food with vegetables and starches is a standard in this country. The trick is to present less fat and more fiber and minerals than the usual American diet, and the key lies with beans and seafood. Most of the dinner recipes provided are built on beans or seafood as a major ingredient.

DESSERTS

What creates a dessert? Sweet taste, a different texture (creamy or crunchy), and a pretty appearance. This can easily be accomplished with sugar and cream, but these ingredients are very low in nutrients. The challenge of dessert is to make it nutritionally rich, supplying, in particular, some vitamins and minerals missing from the remainder of the meal, and, at the same time, being sweet and interesting in texture and appearance. Most "natural food" cookbooks rely on honey for sweetness and vegetable oils or margarine for shortening. This is not substantially different from using sugar and cream (at least cream and butter supply vitamin A). The composition of honey is not much different from sugar, although traces of some minerals and enzymes do remain in honey.

I have approached desserts from the following perspective: The main source of sweetness should be fruits—fresh, dried, puréed, concentrated—because fruits supply some vitamins and minerals that are often not easily obtained elsewhere. Examples: vitamin C in citrus fruits and berries, vitamin A in cantaloupe.

For smooth texture, protein, and additional minerals, either plain yogurt or soft or silken tofu, and for crunchy protein and minerals, nuts and seeds are called for.

Bulk and substance can be provided by whole grains, and eggs can contribute cohesion as well as their own protein and minerals.

For shortening, my preference is a mixture of butter and flaxseed (or walnut) oil. Why? Flaxseed oil is an excellent source of omega-3 EFAs and has virtually no flavor. I do not like flaxseed oil for frying, because it oxidizes rapidly and the EFAs are destroyed. In baking, on the other hand, things are different. A hot oven has lost oxygen and in the interior of a baking bread or pastry there is relatively little oxygen to destroy the oil.

Butter need not be completely avoided by children. It contributes vitamin A and a pleasing flavor to the flaxseed oil.

A word about baking soda and baking powder. These are necessary for certain baked goods such as muffins. They help dough rise. Baking soda is pure sodium bicarbonate; therefore, it adds sodium to the recipe. This is unavoidable and not a major concern if no other salt is added.

Baking powder is a mixture of sodium bicarbonate, calcium acid phosphate (as a stabilizer), and cornstarch. Most baking powders contain sodium aluminum sulfate. Avoid these. Aluminum is a toxic metal that does not belong in anyone's diet, especially a child's. It can accumulate in the central nervous system and contribute to brain dysfunction. Some cases of Alzheimer's disease are thought to reflect susceptibility to toxic accumulation of aluminum in the brain. Check your health-food store for an aluminum-free baking powder, such as Rumford.

Aluminum can also enter food from aluminum cookware. The rate at which aluminum is leached from cookware depends on the acidity of the water and food, the duration of cooking, and the presence of fluoride in the water. A study at the Institute of Fundamental Sciences in Hantana, Sri Lanka, published in the prestigious journal *Nature,* found that 1 part per million (ppm) of fluoride in water released 200 ppm of aluminum when boiled for ten minutes in aluminum cooking pots. That's 1,000 times the amount leached out by nonfluoridated water. Prolonged boiling was capable of tripling the aluminum concentration. Since these concentrations of fluoride are found in municipal water supplies, it seems prudent not to use aluminum cookware with fluoridated tap water. Highly acidic water, found in many wells, and acidic foods, such as tomatoes, also extract considerable aluminum. The only cookware we use in our household is cast iron, glass, or porcelain, and occasionally stainless steel.

STAPLES

In the section below, any products with an asterisk are generally available only in health-food stores. Otherwise, all staples are available either in supermarkets or health-food stores.

Grains and Grain Products

When you purchase grains in the supermarket, make sure the label reads "whole grain," "whole wheat," and so on. For example, Heckers whole wheat flour is a good brand. Good health-food store brands are Arrowhead Mills, Shiloh Farms, Walnut Acres, Erewhon, and Olde Mill. Refrigerate grains for maximum freshness.

Whole wheat flour
    Wheat flakes*
    Whole wheat pastry flour*
    Soy powder
    Soy flour*
    Yellow cornmeal
    Oat flakes
    Rolled oats (Old-fashioned Quaker Oats is fine.)
    Oat bran (Sovex brand of oat bran is available in supermarkets. Or purchase Mother's Oat Bran, which is found in health-food stores.)
    Wheat bran (Wheat bran can be found in bulk in health-food stores. Supermarkets carry miller's bran [unprocessed wheat bran] by Sovex. A good health-food store brand is Shiloh Farms.)
    Brown rice* (Most supermarkets stock long-grain rice. I prefer short-grain in general, although for rice pudding the long-grain is more moist and tender. Purchase short-grain rice in the health-food store.)
    Barley flakes*
    Whole wheat pita bread

Pasta (Pasta comes in many colors and shapes. Experiment as you wish. Supermarket pasta made with semolina flour has slightly more nutrient value than that made with regular processed white flour. Those with added soy flour have more protein value. Whole-grain pasta has the highest nutrient value.)

Dried Beans and Peas

These will keep up to a year. It is not necessary to refrigerate them, unless they are cooked. They will keep cooked in the refrigerator for up to five days. Or store cooked beans in the freezer in meal-size portions. They will keep up to three months. Look for beans that are uniform in size and color so that they will cook evenly. Avoid those that are dull looking, which indicates age, or have tiny pinholes, which indicates insect invasion. If you purchase canned cooked beans, try to find them without added sodium. Goya and Progresso supermarket brands have sodium as well as disodium EDTA and calcium chloride. Eden brand in the health-food store has no chemicals, but has soy sauce, which contains sodium. Rinse all canned beans well before use.

Lentils
Navy beans
Great Northern beans
Pinto beans
Black beans
Black-eyed peas
Kidney beans
Adzuki beans*
Split peas

Oils

Olive oil. Berio is a good brand: light and mild-tasting. If you use olive oil frequently, keep it out of the refrigerator, since olive oil gets thick and cloudy when refrigerated. (It will return to its normal consistency after being left at room temperature for a few minutes.)

Flaxseed oil.* Recently, a Canadian firm, Omega Nutrition, has begun exporting a high-quality flaxseed oil to the United States. It can be found in some health-food stores or may be purchased from Allergy Resources, 62 Firwood Road, Port Washington, N.Y. 11050 or from Omega Nutrition, 165-810 West Broadway, Vancouver, British Columbia V5ZYC9.

Unrefined sesame oil.* Arrowhead Mills, Eden, or Erewhon are good brands.

Walnut oil. Hold on to your seats when you see the price! This is just to be used as a delicious flavoring and for its good nutritional value.

Nut Butters

These should be kept in the refrigerator to avoid rancidity. Be sure your peanut butter has no sugar added. Read the label. Remember that dextrose and corn sweetener are sugars. If you buy it freshly ground, be sure that it is refrigerated right away, since without salt and preservatives it gets rancid quickly.

Peanut butter. Sugar-free supermarket brands: Health Valley, Smuckers Natural. Health-food store brands: Bazzini, Erewhon, Arrowhead Mills.

Sesame tahini. Note that "sesame butter" is different from tahini. Sesame butter is made from roasted sesame seeds and is much thicker in consistency, so it will affect the recipe. Sesame tahini is made from unroasted sesame seeds and is runnier than sesame butter. Good brands of sesame tahini are Near East (available in supermarkets), Arrowhead Mills, Erewhon, and Alyamani Delights, Inc.

Nuts and Seeds

Purchase nuts and seeds from a store with a fast turnover, since nuts and seeds turn rancid quickly. Avoid those that look shriveled, discolored, or moldy. Store nuts and seeds in the refrigerator.

Sesame seeds
Sunflower seeds (hulled)
Pumpkin seeds
Walnuts
Almonds
Filberts
Flaxseed* (Shiloh Farms flaxseed is a good brand.)

Dried Fruit

Purchase unsulfured dried fruit; that is, fruit that has not been treated with the toxic chemical sulfur dioxide to preserve the color and soft texture. Unsulfured dried fruit will be darker and drier, but can be plumped up by soaking in hot water. It can be purchased in the health-food store. Shiloh Farms is a good brand. Dried fruit can be kept in the freezer for months.

Raisins

Black mission figs* (Shiloh Farms brand is good.)

Pitted dates

Dried apples* (If these are sold in bulk, they are much less expensive.)

Seasonings and Flavoring Agents

Apple cider vinegar or rice vinegar

Vanilla and almond extract (Purchase pure extracts with no added artificial color or preservatives. Good brands are Farm Product or Nutriflavors.)

Baking soda

Frozen orange, apple, and pineapple concentrates (Concentrates are used as sweeteners. All frozen concentrates are found in the frozen foods section of the supermarket. They are what you would use to make fruit juice. Use them undiluted in the recipes.)

Honey (Be sure it has no added preservatives. Never give honey to a child who is less than a year old.)

Soy sauce (Be sure it has no MSG, corn syrup, or coloring added. Purchase reduced-sodium soy sauce, if it is available. If your child is allergic to wheat, purchase wheat-free soy sauce. Good brands: Erewhon, Eden, Reduced Sodium Sushi Chef [found in supermarkets].)

Lemon juice (Squeeze fresh.)

Other Staples

Tofu (Tofu comes firm, soft, or silken. Use the kind called for in the recipe. If you can't find silken, use soft. Purchase it packaged in the dairy section of the market. Tofu left sitting in water in the open, or stored in temperatures less than dairy storage, may have bacterial overgrowth. Signs of spoilage are a bulging package and/or a smell like vinegar or sulfur. Store your tofu in the refrigerator in a container of water. Change the water daily. It should keep for three to five days. It will also keep in the freezer for up to two months, but will be spongier and more fragile. A common brand of Tofu is Tomsun.)

Eggs

Milk

Plain yogurt

Frozen fish (Fresh fish is preferable, but it helps to have some frozen on hand for last-minute meals.)

Corn tortillas (To make into crisps [see p. 266]. Purchase those made *only* with corn, water, and lime. They are unbaked and can be found in the freezer section of the supermarket or health-food store. A health-food store brand is Garden of Eatin Corntillas.)

Jams and jellies (Purchase those without any added sweeteners, including honey. Good brands are Polaner All-Fruit, Sorrell Ridge [fruit only], and Just Fruit. Other good sugar-free toppings are Poiret apple-pear spread or a pure apple butter, such as Shiloh Farms.)

Applesauce (Purchase unsweetened applesauce, such as Mott's Natural, Eden, or Cherry Hill applesauce.)

Sugar-free catsup* (A good brand, found in health-food stores, is Westbrae unsweetened "unketchup.")

Flaked coconut (If you purchase it in the supermarket, be sure it is unsweetened. Remember that corn syrup is sugar. Read the label.)

HOW TO OIL A PAN

To use as little oil as possible, put a bunched-up paper towel over the opening of your favorite cooking oil. (Olive oil, such as Berio, is best for cooking.) Tip the bottle quickly upside down, then right-side up. Whatever small amount of oil is on the towel can be used to wipe the pan. Another idea: brush the pan with an oiled pastry brush.

For greasing baking pans for cakes, and so on, a small amount of butter is fine. It contributes vitamin A and a pleasing flavor to the baked goods.

Most baking pans are aluminum or glass, and glass can be hard to find. Using a nonstick-surface pan or lining the inside with wax paper will keep baked goods from sticking and will act as a barrier between the food and the aluminum.

HOW TO COOK BEANS

Beans should be rinsed several times to get rid of grit and other particles.

All beans except lentils, split peas, adzuki beans, baby limas, and black-eyed peas need to be soaked for at least three hours before cooking. (Soybeans and chick-peas require overnight soaking.)

Since beans expand up to three times in volume when moistened, use a pot large enough to accommodate their increased size when you cook them.

Most beans require two to four times liquid to the volume of beans.

To help get rid of the carbohydrate in the bean that causes intestinal gas, throw away the soak water and replace with fresh water to cook the beans. Also, after the first hour of cooking, replace the water again. You'll loose some nutrients but not many.

Although pressure cooking is faster, cooking beans more slowly (in a regular pot, that is) seems to result in greater digestibility.

A simple technique for determining that beans are cooked: Blow on a bean. If the skin pops, it's done.

Eating fresh beans is preferable to eating canned, since canned beans have added sodium. If you purchase canned beans, rinse them well to help get rid of the sodium.

Cooked beans keep up to three months stored in the freezer, and keep in the refrigerator for up to five days.

BREAKFAST: START THE DAY HEALTHY

JEFF'S BLUEBERRY WHOLE WHEAT PANCAKES
My son Jeff devised this recipe while making brunch for friends. It's become a regular Sunday treat.

MAKES EIGHTEEN 4½-INCH PANCAKES

TIME SAVERS: The batter can be prepared the night before, if you like. In fact, it is even better if allowed to sit in the refrigerator for 3 to 6 hours before use. Alternatively, the dry ingredients (flour and soda) can also be premixed and kept in the refrigerator until pancake time. Cooked pancakes can be kept in the freezer and put in the toaster or microwave.

1½ cups whole wheat flour
½ cup soy powder
2 tsp baking soda
1½ cups fresh blueberries (see Note)
2 eggs
1½ cups buttermilk, or plain yogurt
¾ cup water
2 Tb flaxseed or walnut oil

In a large bowl, stir the flour, soy powder, and baking soda until combined. Add the blueberries and mix until berries are coated with flour. In a medium-size bowl, beat the eggs; then add the buttermilk, water, and oil, and blend thoroughly. Add the liquid mixture to the dry, stirring until combined. Don't overstir or beat the batter—a few lumps are not a problem, and too much mixing will result in tough, rubbery pancakes.

Heat a large nonstick frying pan or griddle (see Note), then oil it lightly. Pour ¼ cup of batter on the griddle for each pancake. Let the batter cook until bubbles appear on the surface and the edges look dry and begin to turn lightly brown. Then turn the pancake and cook about 2 minutes more.

If necessary, add small amounts of oil to the griddle in between pancakes.

To keep the pancakes warm, preheat the oven to the warm setting and put the pancakes on a baking sheet in the oven as you go. If you stack the pancakes, put a cloth between them to prevent them from becoming rubbery.

If desired, top with applesauce (such as Mott's Natural Applesauce or an unsweetened health-food store brand), sugar-free jam (such as Sorrell Ridge or Polaner All-Fruit), low-fat yogurt, or any of the sweet toppings on pages 286–87.

Notes: Frozen blueberries do not work as well in this recipe as fresh.

Using a nonstick frying pan or griddle will cut down on the need to use a lot of oil to make the pancakes, and they bake better on this type of surface.

SESAME WAFFLES

MAKES FOUR 7-INCH WAFFLES

TIME SAVER: The batter can be prepared the night before, if you like. In fact, it is even better if allowed to sit in the refrigerator for 3 to 6 hours before use. Cooked waffles can be kept in the freezer and put in the toaster or microwave.

1 cup whole wheat flour
⅓ cup soy flour
1 tsp baking soda
3 Tb sesame seeds
2 eggs
1 Tb flaxseed or walnut oil
1 cup buttermilk
3 Tb water

In a large bowl, sift together the flours and baking soda. Add the sesame seeds. (At this point, I found it was perfect timing to start heating up an electric waffle iron.)

In an electric blender, mix the eggs, oil, buttermilk, and water. Add the liquid ingredients to the dry, stirring with a few quick strokes till just mixed. Don't worry about a few lumps; it's better to underbeat than overbeat.

Lightly oil the waffle iron. Pour on ½ cup batter per waffle. Each waffle takes between 3½ and 4 minutes to cook to a golden brown. To keep the waffles warm before serving, preheat the oven on the warm setting and put them on a baking sheet in the oven. If you stack the waffles, put a cloth between them to prevent them from becoming rubbery.

Top with sugar-free applesauce (such as Mott's Natural Applesauce, or a sugar-free health-food store brand), sugar-free jam (such as Sorrell Ridge or Polaner All-Fruit), low-fat yogurt, or any of the sweet toppings on pages 286–87.

BRAN MUFFINS

These are a great nonsweet muffin. If you need a sweetener, top the muffin with apple butter, apple-pear spread, or a sugar-free jam. Your children can help you coat the raisins with the flour.
MAKES 12 TO 14 MEDIUM-SIZE MUFFINS

2 cups whole wheat flour
¼ cup soy flour
2 tsp baking soda
¼ to ½ tsp ground cinnamon
1 cup wheat bran
¾ cup raisins
1 egg
2 Tb flaxseed or walnut oil
1¼ cups buttermilk
½ cup apple juice concentrate

Preheat oven to 400° F., and lightly oil a muffin pan or 14 paper muffin cups.

In a large bowl, sift together the flours, baking soda, and cinnamon. (If there is any bran residue, add it back into the mixture. The sifting makes the muffins a little lighter; it's not to remove bran.) Stir the wheat bran into the flour mixture, then add the raisins and stir until the raisins are coated with flour.

In a medium-size bowl, beat the egg with a wire whisk, then add the oil and mix well. Add the buttermilk and apple juice concentrate, and beat thoroughly.

Add the liquid ingredients to the dry all at once, stirring with a few quick strokes just until combined. Don't overbeat or the muffins will be tough. Spoon the batter into the lightly oiled pan or muffin cups, filling each almost to the top with batter.

Bake for 20 minutes, or until the tops of the muffins are lightly brown and a cake tester comes out dry when inserted in the center. Let the muffins sit in the pan for about a minute, then carefully turn out onto a wire rack to cool for a few minutes. Serve hot.

APPLE-COCONUT MUFFINS

MAKES 10 MUFFINS

1½ cups whole wheat flour
1 tsp baking soda
½ tsp ground cinnamon
3 Tb flaxseed, ground (to make ¼ cup ground) (see Note)
1 egg
¼ cup melted unsalted butter
¼ cup flaxseed or walnut oil
2 Tb apple juice concentrate
1 cup sugar-free applesauce
½ cup flaked unsweetened coconut

Preheat the oven to 400° F. Lightly oil 10 muffin cups.

In a large bowl, mix the flour, baking soda, cinnamon, and ground flaxseed. In a medium-size bowl, beat the egg, butter, and oil. Then add the apple juice concentrate, applesauce, and coconut, and mix until well blended. Add the wet ingredients to the dry all at once, stirring just until the mixture is moistened. Don't over-beat or the muffins will be tough. Spoon the batter into the muffin cups, filling each two-thirds full.

Bake for 30 minutes, or until the tops are lightly brown. The insides of the muffins will be slightly moist because of the applesauce.

Note: Flaxseed can be ground in a coffee mill or nut grinder.

GRANOLA

MAKES 7 CUPS

3 cups rolled oats
1 cup oat bran
¼ cup sesame seeds
¼ cup flaxseed
½ cup sunflower or pumpkin seeds
1 cup chopped walnuts
½ cup apple juice concentrate
¼ cup flaxseed or walnut oil
1 tsp vanilla
1 tsp ground cinnamon
2 cups raisins
½ cup flaked unsweetened coconut

Preheat the oven to 350° F. and lightly oil two cookie sheets.

Mix oats, oat bran, seeds, and nuts in a large bowl. Combine the apple juice concentrate, oil, vanilla, and cinnamon in a small bowl.

Add the wet ingredients to the dry, stirring until everything is well coated with the oil mixture. Spread the mixture evenly on the two cookie sheets.

Bake for 18 to 20 minutes, or until golden brown. Stir after 10 minutes. Remove from the oven, and add the raisins and the coconut.

Store in an airtight container in the refrigerator. Serve topped with low-fat milk or apple juice.

MUESLI

MAKES 10 CUPS

3 cups rolled oats
3 cups whole wheat or barley flakes
1 cup oat flakes
1 cup oat bran
1 cup sunflower or pumpkin seeds
1 cup chopped hazelnuts or filberts
1 cup raisins
1 cup packed chopped dried apples

Preheat the oven to 400° F.

In a large bowl, combine the rolled oats, whole wheat or barley flakes, the oat flakes, and oat bran. Spread the grains out in a thin layer on 5 ungreased cookie sheets, using 2¼ cups of grain for a 14-inch-square baking sheet. Shake the cookie sheet so that you have an even distribution of grains. Bake for 4 to 5 minutes, stir and turn the grains with a spatula, and bake them for an additional 1 to 2 minutes, until lightly browned. Let them cool, then put them back in the bowl. Add all other ingredients and mix them together.

Store in an airtight container in the refrigerator. Serve with milk or plain yogurt. Add fresh fruit in season.

STIR-FRIED TOFU

4 oz firm tofu
1 Tb olive oil
Sea salt to taste
⅛ tsp paprika

Slice tofu into squares about ½ inch thick. Heat olive oil in a seasoned cast-iron skillet and quickly stir-fry the tofu. Season with sea salt and paprika, and serve.

SCRAMBLED TOFU

4 oz tofu
1 Tb olive oil
⅛ tsp turmeric
Sea salt to taste
⅛ tsp paprika

Mash a piece of firm tofu about 1¼ inches thick. In a skillet, heat the olive oil, and when it starts to sizzle, add the mashed tofu, and, as you would with an egg, scramble the tofu in the pan with a wooden spatula or fork. Add turmeric for color. Season with sea salt and paprika and serve like a scrambled egg.

SUPERNUTRITIOUS MAIN COURSES

LENTIL AND BARLEY STEW
SERVES 6

¾ cup dried lentils
¾ cup whole barley
1½ cups chopped onion
1 cup chopped celery
2 tsp olive oil
6 cups water
½ tsp rosemary
¼ tsp thyme
1 bay leaf
3 cups sliced carrots
3 cups chopped potatoes
Salt to taste
Pepper to taste
1 cup chopped parsley

Put the lentils and barley in a large bowl, and add water to cover. Pour off the water and refill the bowl. Do this several times until the water is clear. Drain and set aside. In a heavy 4-quart pot, sauté the onion and celery in the olive oil until the onion is clear and soft. Add the water, drained barley and lentils, and herbs. Bring stew just to the boil, then turn down the heat, cover, and let simmer over low heat for 15 minutes. Remove the bay leaf from the stew, and add the carrots and potatoes. Continue cooking until the lentils and barley are soft, about 30 minutes, stirring occasionally. When the stew is done, stir in salt and pepper to taste, then add the parsley.

LENTIL-NUT LOAF
This tastes great by itself or with tomato sauce. It's also good cold, by itself or as a sandwich—a great lunch for brown-bagging it to school.
SERVES 6

⅓ cup lentils
1⅓ cups cold water
¼ cup flaxseed
½ cup hot water
2 eggs
½ tsp soy sauce
¼ tsp thyme
¼ tsp rosemary
1 cup chopped onion
1 cup finely chopped celery
¼ cup chopped parsley
¼ cup sesame seeds
1½ cups ground nuts or seeds (sunflower seeds, almonds, or pumpkin seeds)
½ cup whole-grain bread crumbs (see Note)
1 cup chopped walnuts

Rinse the lentils, removing any small stones. Put the lentils in a pot with cold water. Bring the water to a boil, lower the heat, and simmer 50 minutes, or until the lentils are soft.

Meanwhile, prepare the rest of the ingredients for the loaf: Put the flaxseed in a cup with the hot water. The seeds will absorb the water, forming a gel in about 20 minutes. This will help hold the loaf. It will also provide a soft, crunchy texture, and the flaxseeds are high in EFAs.

Preheat the oven to 350° F.

In a large bowl, beat the eggs, then add the remaining ingredients, including the cooked lentils and flaxseed gel.

Press the mixture into a lightly greased 9-by-5-by-3-inch loaf pan. Bake for 1 hour.

Note: Make your own bread crumbs from homemade bread with a food processor or blender, or purchase bread crumbs that have no added sugar, salt, or preservatives.

VEGETARIAN BURGERS

MAKES 10 BURGERS

Divide the mixture into ½-cup portions to form patties that are 3 inches in diameter and 1 inch thick, or any size you like. Place the patties on a lightly greased cookie sheet and bake 15 minutes on each side at 350° F. Enjoy the burgers with sugar-free catsup and a whole-grain bun or pita bread.

SPANISH RICE AND BEANS
MAKES 5 CUPS BEAN MIXTURE AND 7 CUPS RICE

1 cup dried pinto or kidney beans (see Note)
5¾ cups water
2 cups short-grain brown rice
1 garlic clove, crushed
1 cup chopped onion
1¼ cups chopped sweet red pepper
2 tsp olive oil
3½ cups chopped tomatoes
¼ cup tomato paste
1½ tsp ground coriander
½ tsp ground cumin
Salt and pepper to taste

Soak the beans in 4 cups water a minimum of 3 hours. (If it's easier to soak them overnight, do so, but put them in the refrigerator to prevent fermentation.) Discard the soaking water. Add 2½ cups fresh water to the soaked beans and bring to a boil. Reduce heat to a low simmer and cook the beans, covered, for 1½ hours, or until they are soft. Drain them, and set aside.

While the beans are cooking, prepare the rice. Rinse the rice to remove any foreign particles. Put it in a 2-quart pot with 3¼ cups water. Bring just to a boil, stir the rice once, cover, then reduce the heat to a low simmer. Cook for 40 minutes. Try not to lift the lid of the pot, or you'll have soggy rice. Shut the heat off without peeking, and let sit until serving time.

In a large frying pan, sauté garlic, onion, and pepper in olive oil until the onion is clear and the pepper is soft. Add the cooked beans, tomatoes, tomato paste, and seasonings. Stir, and let simmer while you serve the rice. Add salt and pepper to taste. Serve beans over hot rice.

Note: If you prefer to use canned beans, rinse them thoroughly to remove any added sodium or preservatives.

FRIED LIVER ITALIANO

SERVES 6 TO 8

2 eggs
1 cup whole-grain bread crumbs
½ cup grated Parmesan
1 tsp oregano
1 lb beef livers, cut into thin strips or cubes
1 Tb olive oil
1 lb mozzarella, cut into thin slices

Preheat the oven to 500° F. Lightly grease with olive oil a 9-by-13-by-3-inch casserole.

In a medium-size bowl, beat the eggs. Mix the bread crumbs, Parmesan, and oregano in another medium-size bowl. Put the liver pieces in the bowl with the beaten eggs. Take several pieces of the liver out of the egg mixture, shake off any excess egg, then put the pieces into the bowl with the breading mixture. Cover the pieces with the breading, then put them on a plate. Repeat this process, breading several pieces of liver at a time, until all the liver is breaded and set on the plate.

Heat the olive oil in a large frying pan. When the oil is hot but not smoking, put in the liver and let it brown, about 2 minutes. Turn the pieces and repeat on the other side for 1 to 2 minutes more, or until golden brown. Remove from skillet and set aside.

Repeat procedure until all liver pieces are cooked, adding a little more olive oil if necessary. Spread half the liver pieces over the bottom of the oiled casserole. Put half the mozzarella slices over the liver. Add the remaining liver, than another layer of mozzarella.

Put the casserole in the preheated oven. Bake 10 minutes, or until the cheese is melted and a little brown. Serve with whole wheat spaghetti.

VARIATION: Add tomato sauce and a sprinkling of more Parmesan for liver parmigiana.

TROPICAL LIVER

SERVES 4

⅓ cup pineapple juice concentrate
2 Tb soy sauce
1 lb liver, cut into ½-inch cubes
2 tsp butter
1 cup chopped scallions
1 cup chopped walnuts
4 cups cooked brown rice
1 cup chopped fresh or unsweetened canned pineapple chunks,
  juice reserved

Preheat the broiler.

Mix the pineapple juice concentrate and soy sauce in a broiler pan, and add the liver cubes. Set aside.

Melt the butter in a large frying pan. Add the chopped scallions and walnuts. Sauté over low heat until the scallions are soft. Add the rice and chopped pineapple, and sauté for 2 minutes.

Place pan with liver pieces in preheated broiler. Broil for 10 minutes, turning twice. When the liver is done, add it to the rice mixture. Stir until all ingredients are thoroughly combined.

Stir some of the reserved pineapple juice into the broiler juices to make a sauce. Add it to the liver mixture as you wish, or serve separately. (Extra soy sauce can also be added, if necessary, for flavor.)

CHINESE STIR-FRY

This recipe is delicious by itself, or served over brown rice.
SERVES 4

2 Tb unrefined sesame oil
¼ cup chopped scallions
2 tsp finely chopped fresh gingerroot
8 oz hard tofu, chopped, or 1½ cups sliced meat or chicken
1 medium carrot, sliced ¼ inch thick

1 cup sliced broccoli stems
½ cup water chestnuts, sliced in half
2 cups broccoli florets
1 cup snow pea pods, cut in half
¾ cup mung bean sprouts
1 to 1½ tsp soy sauce
1 Tb sesame seeds

Heat the sesame oil in a large frying pan or wok until the oil is quite warm but not hot enough to smoke or sputter. Add the chopped scallions, and sauté till they are soft, about 5 minutes.

Add the ginger, tofu, and carrot. Sauté until the tofu is lightly browned, about 10 minutes. (If you are using meat, you'll need to add it later; otherwise it will be overcooked and tough.)

Push the tofu and carrots to the side of the pan.

Add the broccoli stems and water chestnuts (and meat strips), and sauté 2 minutes, then add the broccoli florets and snow peas. Sauté 2 more minutes, then add the bean sprouts and sauté another 2 minutes.

Add the soy sauce to taste, and sprinkle with sesame seeds.

SEAFOOD RATATOUILLE

Fish can be canned, drained, and flaked tuna or mackerel, or fresh or frozen fillets, such as cod, sole, or flounder. If you use frozen, try to get *deboned* fish. Otherwise, try to remove the bones the best you can. If you are using canned fish such as tuna, use three 8-oz cans of water-packed fish, well drained. Scallops, although not as good nutritionally, are also quite tasty with this recipe.

SERVES 4

¼ tsp oregano
½ tsp basil
¼ tsp thyme
½ tsp rosemary
Freshly ground pepper
1 medium eggplant, peeled and chopped into 1-inch cubes
2 garlic cloves, minced
1½ cups sliced zucchini
1¼ cups chopped onion
1 lb fillets of cod, sole, or flounder
3 large tomatoes, diced
1 green pepper, seeded and diced
Lemon juice to taste
½ cup chopped parsley

Preheat the oven to 375° F.

Mix the herbs and pepper together in a small bowl.

Spread the eggplant cubes over the bottom of an 8¼-by-13-by-3-inch ovenproof pan. Sprinkle half of the minced garlic over the eggplant. Sprinkle half of the herbs and pepper over, then put on a layer of zucchini slices, followed by a layer of chopped onion. Bake for 15 minutes.

Cut the fillets into 1-inch pieces, and set aside.

Remove the eggplant, zucchini, and onion mixture from the oven, and place a layer of fish pieces on top. Sprinkle over the remaining garlic and herb mixture. Add the diced tomatoes and green pepper. Return the pan to the oven and bake another 10 minutes, or until the fish is cooked through. Remove, squeeze lemon juice on top, sprinkle with parsley, and serve.

BOUILLABAISSE

My son Jeff makes this family favorite for us. Any leftover bouillabaisse can be refrigerated up to three days and reheated for a quick meal.

SERVES 6

1¾ cups chopped onions
2 garlic cloves, minced
2 large carrots, sliced

2 Tb olive oil
1 lb cod, haddock, or mackerel fillets, cut into 1-inch pieces
2 large tomatoes, coarsely chopped
½ tsp thyme
1 tsp rosemary
Pinch saffron
2 large potatoes, diced
1 cup water
1 bay leaf
Pepper to taste
*1 lb mixed oysters, clams, scallops, shrimp, and mussels, as
   desired*
¼ to ½ cup parsley sprigs

In a large pot, sauté onions, garlic, and sliced carrots in olive oil,
until the onions are clear. Add fish, tomatoes, and thyme, rosemary, and saffron, and sauté for 5 minutes. Add the potatoes,
water, and a bay leaf. Bring to a boil, reduce heat and cook for
15 minutes. Season to taste with pepper, and remove the bay leaf.
Add the shellfish, cook another 5 minutes, until the shrimp turns
pink.

Sprinkle in parsley sprigs just before serving for a dash of
color. Serve with whole wheat bread cut into thick slices.

OVEN "FRIED" FISH

SERVES 4 TO 5

½ cup milk, or 1 egg, beaten
¼ tsp tarragon
½ cup whole wheat bread crumbs or cornmeal
½ tsp paprika
½ to 1 tsp grated Parmesan
¼ tsp dry mustard
2½ lb fish fillets
Lemon juice to taste
Lemon slices
Sprigs of parsley

Preheat oven to 475° F. Lightly oil a cookie sheet or shallow baking dish large enough to hold the fillets side by side.

In a bowl large enough to dip the fillets, place the milk or egg, add the tarragon, and combine.

In another bowl large enough to dip the fillets, mix the bread crumbs or cornmeal, paprika, Parmesan, and mustard.

Dip each fillet into the liquid mixture, then roll it in the seasoned cornmeal or bread crumbs. Place the fillets on the cookie sheet or in the baking dish. Bake for 7 to 10 minutes, until the fillets turn golden brown and are just done. Squeeze fresh lemon juice on top. Garnish with slices of lemon and sprigs of parsley.

Serve with brown rice and steamed vegetables. If a spread is desired, use the Basic Tofu Spread or Tomato Sauce (see recipes).

POWER PASTA

PASTA PRIMAVERA

This keeps well for two days. Simply put any leftovers in a steamer or double boiler to warm.
SERVES 6

3 Tb olive oil
2 garlic cloves, minced (optional)
3 cups sliced zucchini
2 cups broccoli florets
1 cup asparagus pieces, ½ inch long
2¼ cups chopped yellow squash
1 cup fresh or frozen small spring peas
8 oz linguini or spaghetti
3 cups chopped tomatoes
2 Tb chopped fresh basil, or 1 Tb dried

GARNISHES (optional):
Olive oil
Feta cheese
Grated Parmesan
Tomato Sauce (see recipe)
Oil and vinegar dressing
Freshly ground pepper
Minced garlic

Heat 2 Tb olive oil in a large frying pan or pot. If desired, sauté minced cloves of garlic. Sauté the zucchini, broccoli, asparagus, squash, and peas until they are slightly soft but still crunchy, about 10 minutes.

Break the pasta into thirds. In a large pot of boiling water, place remaining olive oil, and cook the pasta until it is *al dente*.

Drain the cooked pasta and add it to the vegetables. Mix in the tomatoes and basil, and any garnishes you wish. Stir until everything is well mixed and the flavors are blended. Serve hot.

WALNUT PESTO PASTA
MAKES 1¼ CUPS PESTO, TO SERVE 4 (2 CUPS PASTA AND 2
  TABLESPOONS PESTO PER SERVING)

½ cup walnuts
1½ cups fresh basil leaves
¼ cup chopped fresh parsley
2 garlic cloves, minced
½ cup grated Parmesan
½ to ⅔ cup olive oil
1 lb spinach fettuccine
1 Tb olive oil

Grind the walnuts in an electric blender. You may want to leave a few chunks to add a nice texture to the pesto. Add the basil, parsley, garlic, Parmesan, and ½ cup of olive oil to the blender. If necessary, add more olive oil until you have a thick, grainy paste.

In a large pot of boiling water to which you've added 1 Tb olive oil, cook the pasta until it is *al dente*. Drain the cooked pasta, stir in the pesto and mix well.

TOFU-RICOTTA LASAGNA
SERVES 10 TO 12
TIME SAVERS: Use 3 cups prepared tomato sauce. Be sure it has no added sodium, sugar, or preservatives. You can usually find a good sauce in the health-food store. You can also use frozen spinach.

Tomato Sauce
FOR THE TOFU-RICOTTA FILLING
1 lb firm tofu
1 lb part-skim ricotta
1 egg
½ cup grated Parmesan
¼ tsp nutmeg
½ cup chopped parsley

FOR THE VEGETABLE LAYER
4 cups sliced mushrooms
2 tsp olive oil
*1 lb fresh spinach, washed well, drained, and chopped, or one
    10-oz package frozen*

TO FINISH
9 whole wheat lasagna noodles
Olive oil
3 cups shredded part-skim mozzarella
¼ cup grated Parmesan

Make the Tomato Sauce according to the directions on page 264.

TO MAKE THE TOFU-RICOTTA FILLING: Put all the ingredients in an electric blender or food processor, and blend till you have a smooth purée.

TO MAKE THE VEGETABLE LAYER: In a large frying pan, sauté the sliced mushrooms in the olive oil. When the mushrooms are lightly brown, add the spinach and sauté just enough to cook slightly. If necessary, drain the vegetable mixture.

In a large pot of boiling water to which 1 Tb olive oil has been added, cook the noodles until they are nearly *al dente.* Drain them and sprinkle a little olive oil on them to prevent them from sticking together.
　　Preheat the oven to 400° F.

TO ASSEMBLE THE LASAGNA: Lightly oil a 9-by-13-by-2½-inch baking dish. Spread several spoonfuls of tomato sauce on the bottom of the dish, to keep lasagna from sticking. Lay in 3 noodles lengthwise, top with one-fourth of the shredded mozzarella, one-half of the vegetable mixture, one-half of the tofu-ricotta filling, and about one-half of the tomato sauce. Top with 3 noodles, then add the next one-fourth of the shredded mozzarella, the rest of the vegetable mixture, the rest of the tofu-ricotta filling, and finish with the last 3 noodles. Spread the remaining tomato sauce on top, then add the remaining 1½ cups of shredded mozzarella and the grated Parmesan, mixed together.

Bake for 25 to 30 minutes, or until the cheese is lightly browned. Let stand 15 minutes before cutting, and serve hot.

CHILD-PLEASING SALADS

QUICK AND EASY PASTA SALAD
Pastas come in many interesting shapes: penne is a hollow tube with the end cut on the diagonal; rotelle or fusilli are corkscrew-shaped, and so on. It's fun to mix the different shapes, which can be appealing to children.
SERVES 4

8 oz whole wheat pasta
Olive oil to taste
3 cups chopped tomatoes
1 cup loosely packed chopped fresh basil
Black pepper and sea salt to taste

In a large pot of boiling water to which 1 Tb of olive oil has been added, cook the pasta until it is *al dente*. Drain it in a colander, and run it under cold water to cool, then put it in a large salad bowl. Add the tomatoes and basil. Sprinkle with olive oil. Stir. Add freshly ground black pepper and sea salt to taste.

VARIATION: For more protein, add 1 cup chopped mozzarella.

WHITE BEAN SALAD

SERVES 6

¾ cup navy beans
1 large bunch escarole or spinach, washed and chopped
¼ red onion, sliced
½ cup chopped walnuts
Tarragon dressing (see p. 263)

Soak the navy beans in 2 cups hot water for a minimum of 3 hours. Discard the soak water. Put the beans in a 2-quart pot with 2 cups water, and bring just to a boil. Lower heat and simmer for 45 minutes, or until the beans are soft enough to eat, but not so that they fall apart.

Put the chopped escarole and water to cover it in a pot large enough to hold it, and turn on the heat. Stir the escarole constantly for 1 minute, until all pieces are slightly soft, but not wilted.

Put the cooked navy beans, escarole, onion, and walnuts in a large salad bowl. Toss. Add tarragon dressing to taste.

SUPERIOR SOUPS

NAVY BEAN SOUP

SERVES 4

1 cup navy beans
6 cups water
1 cup chopped onion
2 garlic cloves, crushed
1½ tsp olive oil
2 medium carrots, chopped
2 stalks celery, chopped
¼ tsp rosemary
¼ tsp thyme
Pepper and salt to taste

Rinse the beans; soak them in 3 cups of water for a minimum of 3 hours or overnight. Drain, and put them in a large heavy pot. Add 6 cups of water, bring to a boil, lower heat, and simmer, covered, until soft, about 1 hour. (If you like, after 30 minutes, replace the cooking water with an equal amount of fresh water. This helps reduce the gassy effect of the beans.)

Sauté the onion and garlic in the olive oil until soft. When the beans are cooked or nearly cooked, add the onion, garlic, carrots, celery, rosemary, and thyme. Simmer another 10 minutes.

Add pepper and salt to taste.

VARIATION: Add chopped tomatoes and/or tomato paste.

QUICK AND DELICIOUS SPLIT PEA SOUP
MAKES 5 CUPS

1 cup split peas
3¼ cups water
1 cup chopped onion
1 cup chopped celery
1¼ cups sliced carrots

Wash the split peas. Put the water, split peas, onion, and celery in a medium-size pot, bring just to a boil, then turn down the heat. Cover, and simmer over low heat for 40 minutes. Put the soup in the blender and purée till smooth. Then add the sliced carrots and blend briefly, just enough to have bits of carrot in the soup (unless you like it totally smooth). Return the soup to the pot and cook for another 10 minutes. Serve hot.

TASTY SPREADS, DRESSINGS, SAUCES, AND DIPS

BASIC TOFU SPREAD

MAKES ABOUT 1 CUP

8 oz silken or soft tofu
2 Tb lemon juice or vinegar
¼ tsp dry mustard
⅛ tsp minced garlic, or to taste
2 Tb flaxseed or walnut oil, or 1 Tb flaxseed or walnut oil and
*   1 Tb olive oil*

Put the ingredients in an electric blender or food processor and blend until you have a smooth purée.

VARIATION: Add 1 tsp herbs such as chives, dill, or parsley. (This version is good as a topping for baked potatoes.)

TOFU MAYONNAISE

Tofu makes this a high-protein, high-EFA spread that you can feel good about feeding to your children. It is also easier to make than a mayonnaise with eggs. However, don't expect it to taste like egg mayonnaise, or you'll be disappointed. It has its own delicate flavor.

MAKES ABOUT 1¼ CUPS

2 Tb water
⅛ tsp soy sauce
½ tsp apple juice concentrate
Basic Tofu Spread

Add water, soy sauce, and concentrate to the Basic Tofu Spread and mix well.

TOFU SALAD DRESSING

MAKES 2⅓ CUPS

Basic Tofu Spread
¼ cup white or tarragon vinegar
½ cup olive oil
¼ cup flaxseed or walnut oil
2 Tb water
1 tsp tarragon, dill, or parsley

Blend the ingredients together in an electric blender or food processor. For greater tartness, use more vinegar. To make a tarragon dressing, use tarragon vinegar.

NUT BUTTER SPREADS

Smooth nut butters are a little difficult to make unless you have a hand grinder, which works best. However, you can produce a fairly successful nut butter with an electric blender. To make a nut butter, simply grind nuts or seeds in a blender or hand grinder until you have a powder, then gradually add oil until you have a paste.

If you like a chunky nut butter, simply grind for less time. A coarser grind is also less likely to produce oil separation in the nut butter.

If you use a blender, grind 1 cup of nuts or seeds at a time. If you grind too many nuts and seeds at once, you'll put too much stress on the blender's motor, and you won't get a fine powder.

For oils, use olive, flaxseed, and walnut. The amount of oil depends on the type of grinder you have. A good grinder will require less oil; 1 Tb oil per cup of nut or seed meal is usually enough, although you'll probably need more if you use an electric blender. The instructions that follow use an electric blender.

WALNUT BUTTER

MAKES 1 CUP

2 cups walnuts (6½ oz)
1 Tb flaxseed oil
1 Tb walnut oil
   (or 2 TB walnut oil)
1 Tb water

ALMOND BUTTER

MAKES 1½ CUPS

2 cups almonds (10 oz)
1 Tb flaxseed oil
2 Tb walnut or olive oil
   (or 3 Tb walnut oil)
¼ cup water

SUNFLOWER BUTTER

MAKES 2¼ CUPS

2 cups sunflower seeds (10 oz)
1 Tb soy powder
1 Tb flaxseed or walnut oil
1 Tb tahini
2 Tb water

VARIATION: To make nut butters more flavorful, add apple butter, chopped dates, or raisins for sweetness. For taste, texture, and additional vitamins, mix with shredded carrots, alfalfa sprouts, or chopped green pepper.

Note: Keep all nut butters in the refrigerator to prevent rancidity and oil separation.

QUICK SANDWICH SPREAD

MAKES 1 CUP
PREPARATION TIME: 2 minutes

½ cup plain yogurt
½ cup tahini

Mix the two ingredients together in a small bowl or glass jar. Store in the refrigerator; it will keep for several days.

BASIC EGG MAYONNAISE

Be sure that all ingredients are room temperature before starting. If the oil is cold, warm it to tepid (about 70° F.).
MAKES 2½ CUPS

1 egg
¾ tsp dry mustard
1 Tb cider or brown rice vinegar, or lemon juice
1 Tb lemon juice
1 cup olive oil
1 cup flaxseed or walnut oil

Put the egg, mustard, vinegar, and lemon juice in an electric blender. Mix the oils together in a bowl or a 4-cup measuring cup that pours easily. Blend the egg mixture; while the blender is running on a low speed, very slowly pour in the oil mixture in a thin, steady stream. Eventually the mixture will emulsify. Continue adding oil until correct consistency is obtained. (If the mayonnaise separates, remove it from the blender jar, blend another egg in the jar, then slowly pour the mayonnaise back into the jar and blend until correct consistency is obtained.)

Store in the refrigerator in a glass container.

VARIATION: For a dill mayonnaise that is delicious with cold salmon or bean salads, add to the basic mayonnaise 2½ tsp freshly chopped minced chives or the green part of a scallion, and 1½ tsp dry dillweed, or to taste.

BASIC OIL AND VINEGAR DRESSING

This dressing is good for vegetable salads, bean salads, or pasta.
MAKES 1 CUP

¼ cup cider vinegar
½ tsp basil
1 garlic clove, minced
½ cup olive oil
¼ cup flaxseed or walnut oil

Put the vinegar, basil, and garlic in an electric blender. Blend briefly, then add the combined oils slowly.

VARIATION: For a tarragon dressing that is great with beans, use tarragon vinegar and 1 tsp tarragon in place of the cider vinegar and basil.

TAHINI-GINGER DRESSING

This keeps well in the refrigerator. It may thicken with refrigeration; just add more water to thin.

MAKES 1 CUP

1 tsp minced gingerroot
1 tsp finely minced scallion
2 to 3 Tb lemon juice
1 tsp soy sauce
½ cup tahini
⅓ cup water

Place all the ingredients in a blender, adding the water last as needed, and purée until well incorporated.

TOMATO SAUCE

MAKES 3 CUPS
TIME SAVER: Prepare ahead, then freeze in 1-cup freezer bags
   or Pyrex containers.

2 lb plum tomatoes, peeled and chopped
1 medium onion, chopped
3 garlic cloves, minced
1 Tb olive oil
2 tsp dried basil
½ to 1 tsp dried oregano
½ tsp thyme
One 6-oz can tomato paste
3 Tb cooked lentils (optional)

Put the plum tomatoes in a blender or food processor and process to a coarse mixture. In a large heavy pot, sauté the onion and garlic in the olive oil until soft. Add the tomatoes, herbs, and tomato paste, and stir well to combine thoroughly.

For a meatier flavor and a heartier sauce, with more minerals and protein, add the lentils.

Simmer over low heat, uncovered, for at least 30 minutes, stirring occasionally. The longer it cooks, the better it will be.

HUMMUS

MAKES 2¼ CUPS
TIME SAVERS: If you can't face the thought of cooking the beans
   from scratch, use canned chick-peas. However, purchase those

with no added salt or preservatives. If the only brands in your market contain added sodium, rinse them very well (at least 3 times) to wash off as much of the additives as possible.

1 cup chick-peas
4 cups water
⅓ cup lemon juice
2 garlic cloves, minced
⅓ cup tahini
2 Tb flaxseed or walnut oil
¼ tsp chili powder

Soak chick-peas in 3 cups water for 4 hours, or overnight. Discard the water. Bring 4 cups of fresh water to a boil, add the soaked chick-peas, cover, and simmer over low heat for 2 hours, or until soft and easily mashed with a fork. (To help reduce the gassy effect of the beans, replace the cooking water with an equal amount of fresh water after 1 hour of cooking.) Drain the chick-peas, reserving the stock. There should be about 2 cups cooked chick-peas.

Put cooked chick-peas in an electric blender or food processor, add the lemon juice, garlic, tahini, flaxseed oil, and chili powder. Blend slowly, using chick-pea stock as necessary to obtain the desired consistency. Chill. Use as a sandwich spread or dip.

MEXICAN BEAN DIP

MAKES 1¼ CUPS

¼ cup chopped onion
1 garlic clove, minced
2 Tb finely chopped celery
1 Tb olive oil
1½ cups cooked kidney or pinto beans (see p. 248)
¼ tsp soy sauce
Ground cumin and cayenne to taste

Sauté the onion, garlic, and celery in the olive oil. Add the beans and seasonings, and stir until well mixed. Put the ingredients in a blender or food processor and purée until smooth. Serve with warmed tortillas.

TOFU-CARROT-DILL DIP

This dip keeps for several days if refrigerated. It will separate when it is stored; just stir before serving.
MAKES 2 CUPS

2 Tb olive oil
1 Tb flaxseed or walnut oil
2 Tb lemon juice
1 Tb water
1 tsp soy sauce
2 cups sliced carrots
1½ Tb finely chopped scallion, green part only
1 garlic clove, minced
1 tsp dried dillweed
6 oz firm tofu

Place everything except the tofu in a blender or food processor and blend briefly, until carrots are coarsely chopped. Add tofu, blend well, until a fairly grainy texture is achieved. Serve with raw vegetables, pita bread, and Tortilla Chips.

NUTRIENT-DENSE SNACKS AND DESSERTS

TORTILLA CHIPS

Purchase unbaked, unfried corn tortillas, which can be found in packages of twelve in the refrigerated section of supermarkets or health-food stores, made with stone-ground corn and water, or corn and water, treated with lime. Because the corn has been treated with lime (calcium carbonate), they are good sources of calcium. Avoid those with other additives. Ordinary chips are fried in oil (usually partially hydrogenated). Aside from being full of this oil, they are also loaded with harmful breakdown products of the oil from frying. "Natural" chips without preservatives are *worse* in this regard than chips with preservatives.
MAKES 48 TO 96 CHIPS

Twelve 5- or 6½-inch corn tortillas, unbaked and unfried
Sea salt to taste
Garlic powder (optional)
Cayenne (optional)
Italian herbs (optional)

Preheat the oven to 350° F.

Cut the 5-inch tortillas in half, then in half again so you have 4 triangles per tortilla. If tortillas are 6½ inches in diameter, cut them in half again. This will yield 8 chips per tortilla. Place the chips on ungreased cookie sheets and bake for 4 minutes on each side, or until crisp. (Some tortillas are thicker, and will take at least 7 minutes on each side.)

Cool, and sprinkle with sea salt to taste. Or sprinkle with a mixture of garlic powder and cayenne, or garlic powder and Italian herbs. Cool.

QUICK PIZZA

For a pizza crust, use either whole wheat English muffins or whole wheat pita bread. For the topping, use beefsteak tomatoes or plum tomatoes, shredded mozzarella cheese, grated Parmesan, dried oregano, dried or fresh basil, minced garlic (optional; the children may not like it), and olive oil. If you like, add a little variety and a few more vitamins and minerals by including other vegetables, such as sliced zucchini or mushrooms.

MAKES 2 SERVINGS PER WHOLE-GRAIN MUFFIN, OR 4 SERVINGS
PER WHOLE WHEAT PITA.

FOR AN ENGLISH MUFFIN

2 slices tomato, or ½ plum tomato, chopped
3 oz shredded mozzarella
1 tsp grated Parmesan
⅛ tsp dried oregano and ⅛ tsp basil, mixed together
¼ tsp olive oil

FOR A PITA BREAD
3 plum tomatoes, chopped
½ medium zucchini, sliced into thin disks
2 large mushrooms, thinly sliced
½ cup shredded mozzarella
1 Tb grated Parmesan
¼ tsp dried oregano
¼ tsp dried basil
½ tsp minced garlic
1 tsp olive oil

Preheat the oven to 425° F.

Split the English muffin or pita bread in half and put the halves on a cookie sheet. (If you like a dry crust, lightly toast the bread in a toaster or oven before adding the toppings.)

Divide ingredients evenly between muffin halves or pita halves, reserving the olive oil. Drizzle the olive oil on top.

Bake for 10 to 15 minutes, or until the cheese is melted and the tomato is soft. Let cool 5 minutes before serving.

FRUIT SHERBET
MAKES 3 TO 5 CUPS, DEPENDING ON CHOICE OF FRUIT

BASIC INGREDIENTS

½ cup powdered milk, or 1 pkg unflavored gelatin dissolved in
⅔ cup warm orange, apple, or pineapple juice (see Note)
6 oz fruit juice concentrate, such as apple or orange
3 medium ripe bananas, or ¾ lb fresh or frozen blueberries, or
1 lb crushed fresh or canned pineapple (see Note), or ½ lb
fresh or frozen strawberries

BASIC PROCEDURE: Mix the powdered milk or gelatin dissolved in fruit juice with the fruit juice concentrate in a blender or food processor. (For a creamier sherbet, increase the amount of powdered milk.) Add 2 or 3 fruits, as preferred, and blend again for 5 minutes, or until smooth.

Pour into ice cube trays or molds and freeze until firm. If molds are not available, use small paper cups (⅓ cup capacity). Put an ice cream stick (available in some supermarkets or variety stores) in the center.

Notes: Dairy is preferred nutritionally in the sherbet. If a dairy-free sherbet is desired, use the gelatin dissolved in warm fruit juice.

Canned pineapple should have nothing added to it.

BANANA-STRAWBERRY SHERBET
MAKES 3½ CUPS, OR 10 FREEZER POPS

⅔ cup fresh orange juice, or ½ cup water plus 2 Tb orange juice concentrate
1 pkg unflavored gelatin
6 oz frozen orange juice concentrate
3 medium bananas
1¼ cups hulled fresh strawberries, washed

Put the orange juice or water and orange juice mixture in the blender. Add all the other ingredients, and blend until you have a smooth purée. Pour this mixture into 2 ice cube trays or 10 molds. Freeze several hours or overnight, until firm.

To serve, blend the frozen sherbet cubes to make a smooth mixture. Serve in dessert dishes, decorated with a sprig of fresh mint and/or a fresh strawberry. Freezer pops are removed from molds and eaten off the stick.

PINEAPPLE-BANANA SHERBET
MAKES 5 CUPS SHERBET, OR 15 FREEZER POPS

⅔ cup water
⅔ cup orange juice concentrate
3 medium bananas
1 lb pineapple, cubed

Follow the same directions as for Banana-Strawberry Sherbet.

BLUEBERRY-APPLE SHERBET
MAKES 4 CUPS, OR 12 FREEZER POPS

½ cup powdered milk
⅔ cup apple juice, or ½ cup water plus 2 Tb apple juice concen-
    trate
6 oz apple juice concentrate
3 medium bananas
12 oz fresh blueberries

Follow the directions in the master recipe.

YOGURT POPS
MAKES 9 FREEZER POPS

8 to 10 oz frozen orange juice concentrate, or 2 pints fresh
    strawberries or one 20-oz pkg frozen
2 cups plain yogurt or soft or silken tofu

If you use strawberries, purée fresh or frozen berries in a blender,
then add the yogurt or tofu. Transfer to molds and freeze for
several hours or overnight, until firm. Insert ice cream sticks for
handles when pops are semifirm. Unmold to serve.

YOGURT-STRAWBERRY POPS
MAKES 6 TO 7 FREEZER POPS

1 pint strawberries
1 cup plain yogurt
¼ cup apple juice concentrate (optional)

Prepare as instructed in master recipe, using apple juice concentrate if purée isn't sweet enough.

FRUIT ICE
Blend fresh fruit—strawberries, pineapple, or watermelon.
Freeze in an ice cube tray, then blend again until smooth. Serve
in dessert compotes, or refreeze in small paper cups.
    You can also use frozen fruit: a 20-oz pkg of frozen strawber-
ries will yield 2 cups purée.

BANANA ICE

Peel a banana and cut it into chunks. Put the chunks on wax paper and freeze until hard. Put the frozen chunks in a blender and blend until you have a smooth, creamy consistency. Occasionally stop the blender and stir the chunks with a rubber spatula to facilitate blending. If you have a difficult time, add ½ to 1 unfrozen banana or some milk or yogurt.

For a little variation, add vanilla and/or other frozen fruits. A favorite is a mixture of strawberries and banana.

It's fun to make banana splits with the children. Put slices of unfrozen banana in a dessert bowl. Add different kinds of homemade fruit ices and banana ice. Pour a little orange juice concentrate or pineapple juice concentrate over the top, then sprinkle with grated coconut, chopped nuts and seeds, and raisins.

Note: If you own a Champion juicer, it's even easier to make ices. Simply put the frozen fruit through the juicer.

RICE PUDDING

This is a delicious rice pudding that isn't sweet.
SERVES 6

½ cup long-grain brown rice
1¾ cups water
⅓ cup raisins
4 eggs
2½ cups low-fat milk
2 tsp vanilla
½ tsp ground cinnamon, or ¼ tsp grated nutmeg (see Note)

Rinse the brown rice, cleaning it well. Put it and water in a 2-quart pot. Bring the water just to a boil, cover, and turn the heat down very low. Simmer for 50 minutes. The rice should be a little wetter than usual.

Preheat the oven to 350° F.

Put the raisins in a small bowl and add hot water to cover plus an inch. Let the raisins plump for 10 minutes. Lightly beat the eggs, add the milk, vanilla, and cinnamon, if desired. Lightly butter a 2-quart baking dish.

When the rice is cooked, add it to the liquid mixture, and stir, mixing well. Drain the raisins. Stir them into the rice mixture.

Pour the pudding into the buttered baking dish. Bake for 35 to 40 minutes, or until the pudding is set. (It is set when a knife inserted into the side comes out clean. The center may seem too wet still. Don't worry, it will continue to cook and set after you take it out of the oven. Overcooking will cause it to collapse and turn to liquid.)

Sprinkle the top with cinnamon or nutmeg if you haven't added it yet. Let sit a few minutes before serving. Or serve cold.

Note: If you love the taste of cinnamon, add it to the pudding rather than sprinkling it on top.

TOFU CUSTARD

A high-protein, mineral-rich, delicious pudding.

SERVES 4

3 eggs
1 cup firm tofu
2 Tb rice malt sweetener, or ¼ cup honey
1 cup milk
1 tsp vanilla
½ tsp ground cinnamon
⅛ tsp nutmeg (optional)

Preheat the oven to 350° F. Lightly butter a 1½-quart casserole dish.

Beat the eggs in a medium-size bowl. In a blender or food processor, blend the tofu, sweetener or honey, milk, vanilla, and cinnamon until smooth. Pour the blended mixture into the bowl with the beaten eggs, and stir, mixing well.

Pour the custard mixture into the buttered casserole dish. Bake for 1 hour. Sprinkle with nutmeg before serving, if desired.

TOFU-ORANGE PUDDING

SERVES 6

2 cups silken tofu
2 small bananas
½ cup orange juice concentrate
2 tsp vanilla
½ cup buttermilk
Grated orange peel (optional)
Sprig of mint (optional)
Chopped nuts (optional)

Put all the ingredients except optional garnishes in a blender or food processor. Blend until smooth. Pour into individual serving dishes (glass-stemmed dessert dishes look nice). Chill about 1 hour, until a nice pudding texture is achieved.

If you wish, decorate with grated orange peel and a sprig of mint, or sprinkle chopped nuts on top.

AMBROSIA

SERVES 6

4 oranges, peeled and sliced
¾ cup unsweetened shredded coconut
1 Tb orange juice concentrate
⅓ cup pineapple juice, or 1 Tb pineapple juice concentrate mixed with ¼ cup water
Whole strawberry (optional)
Chopped walnuts, sliced almonds, or sesame seeds (optional)

Put the orange slices in a large bowl. Add the coconut and mix thoroughly. In a separate bowl, mix the orange juice concentrate and pineapple juice or pineapple juice concentrate and water. Pour this mixture over the orange slices and coconut. Stir again.

Refrigerate for 1 hour before serving. Put the ambrosia in a glass dessert compote. Top with a whole strawberry, or sprinkle with chopped walnuts, sliced almonds, or sesame seeds.

PEANUT BUTTER CHEWS

These are fun to make with children. "Little hands" can help you
blend the dough by kneading it.
MAKES 24 CHEWS

1½ cups rolled oats
½ cup sunflower seeds
½ cup raisins (see Note)
½ cup peanut butter
½ cup apple juice concentrate

Preheat the oven to 350° F.

Put the rolled oats, sunflower seeds, and raisins in a large
mixing bowl. Mix, then add other ingredients and mix well until
combined. Let the mixture sit a minute so that the oats can soak
up some of the moisture. Meanwhile, lightly oil a cookie sheet.

Shape the dough into tablespoon-size pieces, and put them on
the cookie sheet. Flatten them slightly.

Bake for 12 minutes, or until lightly browned. Let cool on a
wire rack.

Store in an airtight container in the refrigerator. They keep
for several days.

Note: If the raisins are too dry or hard, soak them in hot water
a few minutes to allow them to plump, drain, then use.

SESAME-SPICE OATMEAL COOKIES

It takes lots less time if you have small helping hands to form
these cookies. Making oatmeal cookies is a great opportunity for
fun in the kitchen with your children.
MAKES 100 COOKIES

1 cup pitted dates (8 oz)
1 cup orange juice, or ¼ cup orange juice concentrate plus
  ¾ cup water
¼ cup butter, melted
3 cups rolled oats
1 cup whole wheat flour
½ tsp baking soda

½ tsp ground cinnamon
Pinch of ground cloves
Pinch of grated nutmeg
Pinch of ground ginger
1 cup raisins
1 cup sesame seeds
½ cup flaxseed or walnut oil

Preheat the oven to 350° F. Lightly oil two baking sheets.

Place pitted dates in a medium-size saucepan, and cover with the orange juice or orange juice concentrate and water. Simmer until soft.

In a large bowl, combine the rolled oats, flour, baking soda, and spices.

Add the raisins and sesame seeds to the dry mixture, stirring so that the raisins are covered with flour.

By now the dates should be soft. Put the dates and their liquid, melted butter, and flaxseed or walnut oil in a blender or food processor. Purée until smooth. Pour this mixture into the dry ingredients. Stir until well mixed.

Drop the dough by heaping teaspoonfuls onto the oiled cookie sheets. Bake for 15 minutes, or until cookies are brown around the edges. Cool on a rack.

BANANA-NUT OATMEAL COOKIES
MAKES 24 COOKIES

2 cups rolled oats
½ cup chopped walnuts, pecans, or sunflower seeds
1 cup raisins
3 medium bananas
2½ Tb butter, melted
2½ Tb flaxseed or walnut oil
1 tsp orange juice concentrate

Preheat the oven to 350° F. Lightly butter and flour a baking sheet.

In a large bowl, combine the rolled oats, nuts, and raisins.

Put the bananas, melted butter, oil, and orange juice concentrate in a blender or food processor, and blend until you have a smooth liquid.

Add the liquid mixture to the oat mixture and mix well, until the oats have absorbed the liquid and are fairly soft.

Drop the dough by tablespoonfuls onto the buttered and floured baking sheet, leaving ½ inch between the cookies. They do not spread as they bake, so shape them as you wish them to look. Bake for 20 to 25 minutes, or until brown around the edges. Cool on a rack.

DATE-NUT BARS

These are a chewy newton type of sandwich cookie, with a delicious date filling.

MAKES THIRTY-SIX 1½-INCH-SQUARE BARS

FOR THE FILLING
8 oz pitted dates
½ cup orange juice concentrate
½ cup chopped walnuts

FOR THE CRUST
1½ cups whole wheat flour
1¼ cups rolled oats
*¼ cup ground nuts or seeds, such as almonds, sunflower, flax-
    seed, or walnuts*
1 tsp baking soda
1 tsp ground cinnamon
1 egg
½ cup buttermilk
6 oz orange juice concentrate

Preheat the oven to 400° F. Lightly butter a 9-by-13-by-2-inch baking pan.

TO MAKE THE FILLING: Put the filling ingredients in a medium-size saucepan over low heat, and let them soften for a few minutes. Mash the softened ingredients together until the concentrate is absorbed and you have a spreadable paste. Set aside.

TO MAKE THE CRUST: In a large bowl, combine the flour, oats, ground nuts or seeds, baking soda, and cinnamon. In a small bowl, beat together the egg, buttermilk, and orange juice concentrate. Add the liquid mixture to the dry ingredients. Stir the dough until well mixed.

TO ASSEMBLE THE BARS: Spread half the dough for the crust in the bottom of the lightly buttered pan, using a wet rubber spatula. You may have to moisten the spatula several times in order to spread the dough evenly.

Spread the filling mixture over the crust, also using a moistened rubber spatula. Then top with the remaining crust mixture, again spreading with a wet rubber spatula.

Bake for 30 to 35 minutes. Cut 1½-inch squares with a sharp knife while the bars are warm. Remove them from the pan and let them cool on wire racks. Be careful with the filling; it will be fiery hot.

PUMPKIN COOKIES

MAKES 60 COOKIES

2 eggs
3 oz apple juice concentrate
3 oz orange juice concentrate
2 Tb yogurt
1½ cups pumpkin, either cooked fresh or canned, with no additives
2½ cups whole wheat flour
1 tsp ground cinnamon
½ tsp grated nutmeg
1 tsp baking soda
1 cup raisins
1 cup seeds, such as pumpkin or sunflower, or chopped nuts, such as walnuts

Preheat the oven to 375° F., and lightly oil two cookie sheets.

Put the eggs, juice concentrates, yogurt, and pumpkin in a blender, and purée well. In a large bowl, mix the remaining ingredients, then add the wet ingredients. Stir just until combined but don't overmix or the cookies will be tough.

Drop the dough by tablespoonfuls onto the lightly oiled cookie sheets. These cookies do not spread when baked, so shape the dough as you wish—either in balls, or flattened slightly.

Bake in the preheated oven for 15 to 18 minutes, or until puffed and browned. Cool on a rack.

GRANOLA BARS

Once you've made your granola, these bars are a snap. The longer you keep them, the better they are. Two to three days after making them, they're even better than they are fresh.

MAKES FORTY-EIGHT 1¼-INCH-SQUARE BARS

3 eggs
3 Tb apple juice concentrate
1 tsp ground cinnamon
3 cups Granola (see p. 244)
½ to 1 cup raisins (see Note)

Preheat the oven to 350° F.

In a large bowl, beat together the eggs, apple juice concentrate, and cinnamon. Add the granola and raisins, and mix well. Let the mixture sit in order to absorb some moisture while you lightly oil a 9-inch-square baking pan. Spread the mixture evenly in the pan, and pat it down with the back of a large spoon.

Bake for 25 minutes, or until set and lightly brown around the edges. While the mixture is still warm, cut into 1¼-inch squares. Store in the refrigerator.

Note: If your granola contains raisins, use only ½ cup additional; if it has no raisins, use 1 cup raisins.

FRUIT AND NUT TREATS

MAKES 45 DIME-SIZE PATTIES

⅓ cup pitted dates (about 18)
⅓ cup black mission figs (about 8), stems cut off

3 Tb orange juice concentrate
2 Tb hot water
2¼ cups ground almonds and walnuts
⅓ cup ground flaxseed (see Note)

Put the dried fruit, orange juice concentrate, and hot water in a medium-size bowl. Mash the ingredients with a potato masher or a wooden spoon, until you have a fairly smooth mixture. (A few lumps are fine.)

Combine the nuts and seeds in a small bowl. Remove ½ cup of this mixture and set aside in a cup. (You will use this mixture to coat the patties.)

Add the remaining mixture to the fruit and liquid mixture, and mix well. To form the treats, take a small ball of dough and press it flat slightly to make a dime-size pattie. Put the pattie in the cup of ground nuts and seeds and coat thoroughly.

Keep the patties in a sealed container in the refrigerator.

Note: Flaxseed may be ground in a coffee grinder or nut and seed grinder.

VARIATION: A ½-cup portion of the mixture can be removed before forming the patties, and 2 Tb shredded coconut and ¼ tsp almond extract can be added to it.

NUT BUTTER–COCONUT TREATS
MAKES 40 CANDIES

1 cup peanut or walnut butter, or ¾ cup peanut butter and
  ¼ cup walnut butter
¾ cup chopped raisins, dates, or figs
1½ cups unsweetened shredded coconut
½ cup ground nuts and seeds, such as walnuts, sunflower
  seeds, and flaxseed

In a medium-size bowl, mix the nut butter, dried fruit, and coconut. Make small balls or quarter-size patties. Roll them in the ground nuts and seeds. Keep in the refrigerator.

BASIC SPICE BREAD

This dessert bread recipe is also the basis for a banana or carrot bread. Plus, the bread recipe can be made into a cake with a minor change.

MAKES ONE 6-BY-10-INCH LOAF

1½ cups whole wheat pastry flour
½ cup soy flour
1 tsp baking soda
2 tsp ground cinnamon
¼ tsp grated nutmeg
¼ tsp ground allspice
½ cup raisins
½ cup chopped walnuts
½ cup sesame seeds
3 eggs
¾ cup plain yogurt
¼ cup butter, melted
¼ cup flaxseed or walnut oil
¾ cup orange juice concentrate

Preheat oven to 350° F. Lightly butter a 6-by-10-inch loaf pan.

In a large bowl, sift together the flours, baking soda, and spices. Then add the raisins, walnuts, and sesame seeds. Mix until they are coated with flour to prevent them from sinking to the bottom of the dough.

In another large bowl, beat the eggs, yogurt, melted butter, oil, and orange juice concentrate until they are blended. Stir the liquid ingredients into the dry, blending but not beating.

Pour into the prepared pan and bake for 40 minutes.

SPICE CAKE

MAKES 1 BUNDT CAKE (ABOUT 12 SERVINGS)

To make a cakelike texture, simply substitute 1 egg plus 3 egg whites for the 3 eggs. Beat the whites in a small bowl until they are stiff, then gently fold them into the final batter. Use a Bundt pan in place of the rectangular loaf pan. The Bundt pan gives the appearance of a cake. Top with a frosting after the cake has cooled slightly. See pages 284–85 for frosting recipes.

BANANA BREAD

MAKES ONE 6-BY-10-INCH LOAF

Make the following changes to the Basic Spice Bread recipe:

Substitute ½ cup orange juice concentrate for the ¾ cup
Substitute ¼ cup yogurt for the ¾ cup
Substitute ½ tsp ground allspice for the ¼ tsp
*Add 1½ cup mashed bananas (5 small or 2 to 3 medium) to the
liquid ingredients*

Put the liquid ingredients in a blender instead of in a small bowl
and blend until smooth. Then add the moist ingredients to the
flour mixture and mix as directed.

Pour into the prepared pan and bake at 350° F. for 1 hour.

CARROT BREAD

MAKES ONE 6-BY-10-INCH LOAF

Make the following changes to the Basic Spice Bread recipe:

Substitute ½ cup orange juice concentrate for the ¾ cup
Substitute ¼ cup yogurt for the ¾ cup
Substitute ½ tsp ground allspice for the ¼ tsp
*Add 2½ cups grated carrots (about 9 oz) to the liquid ingredi-
ents*

Pour the batter into the prepared pan, and bake at 350° F. for 1
hour.

CARROT CAKE

Use the same ingredients as the Carrot Bread, except for the
eggs. To lighten the bread to a cakelike consistency, use 1 egg
plus 3 egg whites, beaten till stiff. Use a buttered Bundt pan to
bake the cake. Bake at 350° F. for 1 hour. Let cool, then top with
frosting, such as the Coconut Tofu Frosting on page 285.

PUMPKIN PIE

This pie is denser than most pumpkin pies, but the texture is very
good when served cold. If you prefer a lighter pie, however, add
the optional egg whites.

MAKES 6 SERVINGS

FOR THE PASTRY CRUST

1¼ cups whole wheat pastry flour
8 Tb (1 stick) cold butter
2 Tb flaxseed or walnut oil
1 egg (optional)
Cold water (optional)

FOR THE FILLING

2 cups cooked fresh or canned pumpkin
8 oz firm tofu
3 Tb apple juice concentrate
1 tsp vanilla
2 tsp ground cinnamon
½ tsp ground allspice
4 Tb honey
2 egg whites (optional)

TO MAKE THE PASTRY CRUST: Preheat the oven to 425° F. Put the flour into a medium-size bowl. Cut the butter into 8 pieces, and add them to the flour. Use your fingers to blend the butter into the flour, or cut it in with a pastry blender, until it resembles coarse crumbs. Sprinkle the oil into the flour and butter mixture as you work. Do not overmix, or you'll have a tough crust.

For a flakier crust, beat the egg in a small bowl, then add it to the pastry mixture. Stir it in quickly and lightly with a fork.

Form the dough into a ball. If it is too dry, add a little cold water. Roll out the dough into a 10-inch circle on lightly floured wax paper with a lightly floured rolling pin. (To prevent the wax paper from slipping as you roll, sprinkle a little water under it on your countertop.)

Turn the wax paper over onto a 9-inch pie plate so that the rolled crust falls into the pie plate. Crimp the edges, and prick the bottom of the crust in several places with a fork, to prevent the crust from bubbling up when it bakes. Bake it for 8 to 10 minutes, or until it is lightly browned.

Lower the heat to 350° F., then prepare the filling.

TO MAKE THE FILLING: Place all filling ingredients except the egg whites in a blender, and blend well. If you are adding the egg whites for a lighter texture, beat them in a small bowl until stiff.

Pour the filling mixture into a large bowl, then fold in the egg whites.

Pour the filling into the baked pie shell. Bake for 40 minutes. Refrigerate before serving.

SMOOTHIES

MAKES 2 CUPS

All smoothies must include the following, to provide essential nutrients: 3 Tb yogurt or tofu, 1 small banana, and 1 Tb flaxseed or walnut oil. Note that when using tofu, silken tofu works the best, but firm and soft tofu are also satisfactory. Blend all ingredients in a blender or food processor until you have a smooth drink. You can also freeze the mixtures in molds to make freezer pops.

Following are 5 different delicious smoothies:

ALMOND-YOGURT

10 almonds
½ cup water
3 Tb yogurt
1 small banana
1 Tb orange juice concentrate
1 Tb flaxseed or walnut oil

Grind the almonds in the blender, then add all the remaining ingredients and liquefy.

WALNUT-ORANGE

1 oz walnuts
1 Tb orange juice concentrate
½ cup water
1 small banana, or 5 pitted dates
1 tsp coconut
3 Tb yogurt
1 Tb flaxseed or walnut oil

Grind the walnuts in the blender, then add all the remaining ingredients and liquefy.

TOFU-FIG

3 Tb tofu (1½ oz)
1 small banana
4 black mission figs
1 Tb orange juice concentrate
¾ cup water
1 Tb flaxseed or walnut oil
1 Tb oat bran

Blend all ingredients together in a blender.

PINEAPPLE-TOFU

½ cup pineapple juice, or 1 Tb pineapple juice concentrate and
*   ½ cup water*
1 egg, or 3 Tb tofu
1 small banana
1 Tb flaxseed or walnut oil
3 Tb yogurt
1 cup strawberries (optional)

Blend all ingredients together in a blender.

TAHINI-BANANA

1 Tb tahini
1 small banana
3 Tb tofu
1 Tb flaxseed or walnut oil
2 Tb pineapple juice concentrate
⅔ cup water

Blend all ingredients together in a blender.

GOOD-FOR-YOU FROSTINGS AND TOPPINGS

VANILLA TOFU FROSTING

The ground, soaked flaxseed in the frosting provides nutritional
value and helps hold the frosting together. It will also add little

brown specks to the frosting. If you cannot get or make ground flaxseed, just eliminate. The frosting will still hold very well without it.

MAKES ¾ TO 1 CUP, ENOUGH TO COAT THINLY TOP AND SIDES
OF ONE 9-INCH CAKE

6 oz firm tofu
2 tsp ground flaxseed soaked in 2 tsp water (optional)
2 tsp lemon juice
3 Tb apple juice concentrate
1 tsp vanilla

Put the tofu in a blender and mash lightly with a rubber spatula. Add the other ingredients and blend until you have a smooth frosting. (It should be neither runny nor stiff.) Refrigerate, covered, to thicken further. It can be spread with a rubber spatula before or after refrigeration.

ORANGE TOFU FROSTING

6 oz firm tofu
2 tsp ground flaxseed soaked in 2 tsp water
3 Tb orange juice concentrate
1 oz banana
Grated orange peel

Follow instructions in the master recipe for preparing the frosting, reserving the grated orange peel. Top frosted cake or muffins with the grated orange peel for additional color and vitamin C.

COCONUT TOFU FROSTING

6 oz firm tofu
2 tsp ground flaxseed soaked in 2 tsp water
3 Tb pineapple juice concentrate
1 oz banana
3 Tb coconut
Grated coconut

Follow instructions in the master recipe for preparing the frosting. Top frosted cake or muffins with more coconut, if you like.

PANCAKE AND WAFFLE TOPPINGS

Delicious toppings can be prepared from fresh, frozen, canned, or dried fruits. If a fruit is dry or not very sweet, 2 tsp of fruit concentrate can be added to the mixture to sweeten and moisten it. Orange, apple, or pineapple concentrates are available in supermarkets. You can use canned, crushed pineapple, but be certain it has no sugar syrup or other kinds of sweeteners. If you use frozen fruits, be sure there is no added sugar, corn syrup, or other additives. To use frozen fruit, remove it from the freezer the night before, and let it defrost overnight in the refrigerator. Note that frozen fruits often have a different taste and consistency from fresh—blueberries, for example, are usually smaller and sometimes less tasty.

FRESH FRUIT SPREAD

Blueberries, raspberries, peaches, apricots, apples, papaya, strawberries, or pineapple
⅓ banana (optional)
2 Tb yogurt (optional)
2 Tb applesauce (optional)
2 tsp grated coconut (optional)
¼ tsp ground cinnamon (optional)
2 tsp fruit concentrate (optional)

Blend fresh or frozen fruit in a blender or food processor. One cup of fruit will yield about ½ cup purée. If you like a chunky sauce, don't run the blender very long; if you want a thicker sauce, add the banana. Any of the remaining ingredients can be added to enhance the flavor of the spread.

Try the following variations, or devise your own.

PEACH AND BANANA
MAKES ¾ CUP, ENOUGH FOR 4 TO 6 PANCAKES

½ large banana
1 ripe peach, peeled and pitted
¼ tsp ground cinnamon

Put all the ingredients in a blender, and blend until you have a smooth sauce.

CINNAMON APPLESAUCE
MAKES ¾ CUP, ENOUGH FOR 4 TO 6 PANCAKES

¼ tsp ground cinnamon
¾ cup unsweetened applesauce

Mix the cinnamon into the applesauce. If you like a warm topping, heat the mixture about 1 minute.

YOGURT-TAHINI SYRUP
MAKES ⅔ CUP

¼ cup tahini
¼ cup yogurt
½ tsp ground cinnamon
1 Tb water
1 Tb apple juice concentrate

Stir the ingredients together in a small bowl until they are well mixed.

References

CHAPTER 1: THE VITAL LINK

1. A. S. Kozlovsky et al., "Effects of Diets High in Simple Sugars on Urinary Chromium Losses," *Metabolism* 35 (1986):515–18.

2. D. Toth, "Actual New Cancer-Causing Hydrazines, Hydrazides, and Hydrazones," *Journal of Cancer Research and Clinical Oncology* 97 (1980):97–108. B. Toth and J. Erickson, "Reversal of the Toxicity of Hydrazine Analogues by Pyridoxine Hydrochloride," *Toxicology* 7 (1977):31–36.

3. R. A. Shakman, "Nutritional Influences on the Toxicity of Environmental Pollutants," *Archives of Environmental Health* 28 (1974):105–13.

4. L. Galland, "Increased Requirements for Essential Fatty Acids in Atopic Individuals: A Review with Clinical Descriptions," *Journal of the American College of Nutrition* 5 (1986):213–28.

5. M. S. Manku et al., "Reduced Levels of Prostaglandin Precursors in the Blood of Atopic Patients: Defective Delta-6-

Desaturate Function as a Biochemical Basis for Atopy," *Prosta-glandins, Leukotrienes in Medicine* 9 (1982):615–28. M. S. Manku et al., "Essential Fatty Acids in the Plasma Phospholipids of Patients with Atopic Eczema," *British Journal of Dermatology* 110 (1984):643–48.

6. R. E. Rocklin et al., "Altered Arachidonic Acid Content in Polymorphonuclear and Mononuclear Cells from Patients with Allergic Rhinitis and/or Asthma," *Lipids* 21 (1986):17–20.

CHAPTER 2: PREGNANCY

1. L. Tallarigo et al., "Relation of Glucose Tolerance to Complications of Pregnancy in Non-Diabetic Women," *New England Journal of Medicine* 315 (1987):989–92.

2. S. Monarca et al., "Mutagenicity Assessment of Different Drinking Water Supplies Before and After Treatments," *Bulletin of Environmental and Contamination Toxicology* 34 (1985):815–23.

3. J. E. Blundell and A. J. Hill, "Paradoxical Effects of an Intense Sweetener (Aspartame) on Appetite," *Lancet* 1 (1986):1092–93. S. D. Stellman and L. Garfinkel, "Artificial Sweetener Use and One-Year Weight Change Among Women," *Preventive Medicine* 15 (1986):195–98.

4. M. Stjernfeldt et al., "Maternal Smoking During Pregnancy and Risk of Childhood Cancer," *Lancet* 1 (1986):1350–53.

5. C. Burchfield et al., "Passive Smoking in Childhood," *American Review of Respiratory Diseases* 133 (1986):966–70. Y. Chen et al., "Influence of Passive Smoking on Admissions for Respiratory Illness in Early Childhood," *British Medical Journal* 293 (1986):303–307.

6. K. Simmer, "Are Iron Folate Supplements Harmful?" *American Journal of Clinical Nutrition* 45 (1987):122–25.

7. R. M. McClain and J. M. Rohrs, "Potentiation of the Teratogenic Effects and Altered Disposition of Diphenylhydrantoin by Diet," *Toxicology and Applied Pharmacology* 77 (1985):86–93.

8. A. Conradt et al., "Magnesium Therapy Decreased the Rate of Intrauterine Fetal Retardation, Premature Rupture of Membranes, and Other Complications of Pregnancy," *Magnesium* 4 (1985):20–28.

9. See Note 6 in this chapter.

10. L. J. Taper et al., "Zinc and Copper Retention During Pregnancy: The Adequacy of Prenatal Diets With and Without Dietary Supplementation," *American Journal of Clinical Nutrition* 42 (June 1986):1184–92.

11. G. Saner et al., "Hair Manganese Concentrations in Newborns and Their Mothers," *American Journal of Clinical Nutrition* 41 (1985):1042–44.

12. R. W. Smithells et al., "Further Experience of Vitamin Supplementation for Prevention of Neural Tube Defect Recurrences," *Lancet* 1 (1983):1027–31. M. J. Seller, "Periconceptual Vitamins and Neural Tube Defects," *Lancet* 1 (1985):1392–93. J. Wild et al., "Recurrent Neural Tube Defects, Risk Factors, and Vitamins," *Archives of Diseases in Childhood* 61 (1986):440–49.

13. S. Heller et al., "Vitamin B Status in Pregnancy," *American Journal of Clinical Nutrition* 26 (1973):1339–48.

14. K. Schuster et al., "Effect of Maternal Pyridoxine Hydrochloride Supplementation on the Vitamin B-6 Status of Mother and Infant and on Pregnancy Outcome," *Journal of Nutrition* 114 (1984):977–88.

15. J. Ellis, "Vitamin B-6 Deficiency in Patients with a Clinical Syndrome Including the Carpal Tunnel Defect: Biochemical and Clinical Response to Therapy with Pyridoxine," *Research Communications in Chemical Pathology and Pharmacology* 13 (1976):743–50. J. Ellis, "Clinical Results of a Crossover Treatment with Pyridoxine and Placebo of the Carpal Tunnel Syndrome," *American Journal of Clinical Nutrition* 32 (1979):2040–47.

16. J. Marks, "Critical Appraisal of the Therapeutic Value of Alpha-Tocopherol," *Vitamins and Hormones* 20 (1962):573–98.

17. J. Bell et al., "Perinatal Dietary Supplementation with a Soy Lecithin Preparation: Effects on Development of Central Catecholaminergic Neurotransmitter Systems," *Brain Research Bulletin* 17 (1986):189–95.

18. H. Kondo et al., "Presence and Formation of Cobalamin Analogues in Multivitamin-Mineral Pills," *Journal of Clinical Investigation* 70 (1982):889–98.

19. J. A. Mader and I. A. MacDonald, "Potential Mutagenic Activity of Some Vitamin Preparations in the Human Gut," *Applied and Environmental Microbiology* 48 (1984):902–904.

CHAPTER 3: FROM BIRTH TO SIX MONTHS

1. J. Kumpulainen et al., "Formula Feeding Results in Lower Selenium Status than Breast Feeding or Selenium-Supplemented Formula Feeding: A Longitudinal Study," *American Journal of Clinical Nutrition* 45 (1987):49–53.

2. S. Mann and M. F. Picciano, "Influence of Maternal Selenium Status on Human Milk Selenium Concentration and Glutathione Peroxidase Activity," *American Journal of Clinical Nutrition* 46 (1987):101–109.

3. R. S. Zeiger et al., "Effectiveness of Dietary Manipulation in the Prevention of Food Allergy in Infants," *Journal of Allergy and Clinical Immunology* 78 (1986):224–38.

4. J. Azuma, "Apparent Deficiency of Vitamin B-6 in Typical Individuals Who Commonly Serve as Normal Controls," *Research Communications in Chemical Pathology and Pharmacology* 14 (1976):343–46.

5. L. Styslinger and A. Kirksey, "Effects of Different Levels of Vitamin B-6 Supplementation on Vitamin B-6 Concentrations in Human Milk and Vitamin B-6 Intakes of Breast-Fed Infants," *American Journal of Clinical Nutrition* 41 (1985):21–31.

6. P. A. Schneider, "Breast Milk Jaundice in the Newborn: A Real Entity," *Journal of the American Medical Association* 255 (1986):3270–74.

7. M. Freundlich et al., "Infant Formula as a Cause of Aluminum Toxicity in Neonatal Uraemia," *Lancet* 2 (1985):527–29.

8. P. J. Collipp et al., "Manganese in Infant Formulas and Learning Disability," *Annals of Nutrition and Metabolism* 27 (1983):488–94.

CHAPTER 4: SIX MONTHS TO A YEAR

1. R. S. Zeiger et al., "Effectiveness of Dietary Manipulation in the Prevention of Food Allergy in Infants," *Journal of Allergy and Clinical Immunology* 78 (1986):224–38.

2. E. Pollitt et al., "Iron Deficiency in Behavioral Development in Infants and Preschool Children," *American Journal of Clinical Nutrition* 43 (1986):555–65.

3. W. S. Watson et al., "Oral Absorption of Lead and Iron," *Lancet* 2 (1980):236–37.

4. M. Fulton et al., "Influence of Blood Lead on the Ability and Attainment of Children in Edinburgh," *Lancet* 1 (1987):1221–25.

5. E. Charney et al., "Childhood Lead Poisoning: A Controlled Trial of the Effect of Dust Control Measures on Blood Lead Levels," *New England Journal of Medicine* 309 (1983):1089–93.

6. A. Kahn et al., "Insomnia and Cow's Milk Allergy in Infants," *Pediatrics* 76 (1985):880–84.

7. L. Galland, "Increased Requirements for Essential Fatty Acids in Atopic Individuals: A Review with Clinical Descriptions," *Journal of the American College of Nutrition* 5 (1986):213–28.

8. A. Cant et al., "Egg and Cow's Milk Hypersensitivity in Exclusively Breast-Fed Infants with Eczema, and Detection of Egg Protein in Breast Milk," *British Medical Journal* 291 (1985):932–34.

CHAPTER 5: AGES ONE TO FIVE

1. H. J. Roberts, "Potential Toxicity Due to Dolomite and Bone Meal," *Southern Medical Journal* 76 (1983):556–59.

2. M. Bondestam et al., "Subclinical Trace Element Deficiency in Children with Undue Susceptibility to Infection," *Acta Pediatrica Scandinavica* 74 (1985):515–20.

3. F. A. C. S. Campos et al., "Effect of an Infection on Vitamin A Status of Children as Measured by the Relative Dose Response (RDR)," *American Journal of Clinical Nutrition* 46 (1987):91–94.

CHAPTER 6: NUTRITIONAL FIRST AID TO FIGHT ILLNESS

1. R. Anderson et al., "The Effects of Increasing Weekly Doses of Ascorbate on Certain Cellular and Humoral Immune Functions in Normal Volunteers," *American Journal of Clinical Nutrition* 33 (1980):71–76.

2. F. A. C. S. Campos, "Effect of an Infection on Vitamin A Status of Children as Measured by the Relative Dose Response (RDR)," *American Journal of Clinical Nutrition* 46 (1987):91–94.

3. C. B. Pinnock et al., "Vitamin A Status in Children Who Are Prone to Respiratory Tract Infections," *Australian Pediatric Journal* 22 (1986):95–98.

4. A. M. El-Hfny, *"Candida Albicans* as an Important Respiratory Allergen in the United Arab Republic," *Acta Allergoligica* 23 (1968):297–302. G. Holti, *"Candida* Allergy," in *Symposium on Candida Infections,* ed. H. I. Winner and R. Hurley (London: E. & S. Livingstone Ltd., 1966):73–81. I. H. Itkin and M. Dennis, "Bronchial Hypersensitivity to Extract of *Candida Albicans,"* *Journal of Allergy* 37 (1966):187–94. A. Liebeskind, *"Candida Albicans* as an Allergenic Factor," *Annals of Allergy* 20 (1962):394–96.

5. K. Iwata, "Toxins Reproduced by *Candida Albicans,"* *Contributions in Microbiology and Immunology* 4 (1977):77–85.

6. C. O. Truss, "Tissue Injury Induced by *Candida Albicans:* Mental and Neurologic Manifestations," *Journal of Orthomolecular Psychiatry* 7 (1978):17–37. C. O. Truss, "The Role of *Candida Albicans* in Human Illness," *Journal of Orthomolecular Psychiatry* 10 (1981):228–38.

7. S. Wright and J. L. Burton, "Oral Evening Primrose Seed Oil Improves Atopic Eczema," *Lancet* 2 (1982):1120–22.

8. Consensus Conference—National Institute of Allergy and Infectious Diseases (NIAID) and National Institute of Child Health and Human Development (NICHHD), "Defined Diets and Childhood Hyperactivity," *Journal of the American Medical Association* 248 (1982):290–94.

9. I. C. Menzies, "Disturbed Children: The Role of Food and Chemical Sensitivities," *Nutrition and Health* 3 (1984):39–54.

10. R. Gittelman and B. Eskenazi, "Lead and Hyperactivity Revisited: An Investigation of Non-Disadvantaged Children," *Archives of General Psychiatry* 40 (1983):827–33.

11. J. Egger et al., "Controlled Trial of Oligoantigenic Treatment in the Hyperkinetic Syndrome," *Lancet* 1 (1985):540–45. J. A. O'Shea and S. F. Porter, "Double-Blind Study of Children with Hyperkinetic Syndrome Treated with Multiallergen Extract Sublingually," *Journal of Learning Disabilities* 14 (1981):189–91, 237. E. C. Hughes et al., "Food Sensitivity in Attention-Deficit Disorder with Hyperactivity (ADD/HA): A Procedure for Differential Diagnosis," *Annals of Allergy* 49 (1982):276–80.

12. See Note 11 in this chapter, Hughes citation.

CHAPTER 7: AGES FIVE TO TWELVE

1. R. A. Shakman, "Nutritional Influences on the Toxicity of Environmental Pollutants," *Archives of Environmental Health* 28 (1974):105–13.

2. E. Pollitt et al., "Iron Deficiency in Behavioral Development in Infants and Preschool Children," *American Journal of Clinical Nutrition* 43 (1986):555–65.

3. C. A. Clemetson, "Histamine and Ascorbic Acid in Human Blood," *Journal of Nutrition* 110 (1980):662–68.

4. R. D. Reynolds and C. L. Natta, "Depressed Plasma Pyridoxal Phosphate Concentrations in Adult Asthmatics," *American Journal of Clinical Nutrition* 41 (1985):684–88.

5. R. Anderson et al., "The Effects of Increasing Weekly Doses of Ascorbate on Certain Cellular and Humoral Immune Functions in Normal Volunteers," *American Journal of Clinical Nutrition* 33 (1980):71–76.

6. F. A. C. S. Campos, "Effect of an Infection on Vitamin A Status of Children as Measured by the Relative Dose Response (RDR)," *American Journal of Clinical Nutrition* 46 (1987):91–94.

CHAPTER 8: AGES THIRTEEN TO SEVENTEEN

1. E. W. Rosenberg and B. S. Kirk, "Acne Diet Reconsidered," *Archives of Dermatology* 117 (1981):193–95. A. V. Ratnam and K. Jayaraju, "Skin Diseases in Zambia," *British Journal of Dermatology* 101 (1979):449–53. E. Bendiner, "A Disastrous Trade-Off: Eskimo Health for White Civilization," *Hospital Practice* 9 (1974):156–89.

2. B. L. Snider and D. F. Dieteman, "Pyridoxine Therapy for Premenstrual Acne Flare," *Archives of Dermatology* 110 (1974):130–31.

3. S. Ayres, Jr., and R. Mihan, "*Acne Vulgaris* and Lipid Peroxidation: New Concepts in Pathogenesis and Treatment," *International Journal of Dermatology* 17 (1978):305–11.

4. G. Michaelsson et al., "Serum Zinc and Retinol-Binding Protein in Acne," *British Journal of Dermatology* 96 (1977):283–90. G. Michaelsson et al., "A Double-Blind Study of the Effect of Zinc and Oxytetracycline in *Acne Vulgaris*," *British Journal of*

Dermatology 97 (1977):561–66. G. Michaelsson et al., "Effects of Oral Zinc and Vitamin A in Acne," *Archives of Dermatology* 113 (1977):31–36.

5. S. L. Gortmaker et al., "Increasing Pediatric Obesity in the United States," *American Journal of the Diseases of Children* 141 (1987):535–40.

6. A. J. Wittwer et al., "Nutrient Density—Evaluation of Nutritional Attributes of Food," *Journal of Nutrition Education* 9 (1977):26–30, 198.

7. S. Dalvitt-McPhillips, "A Dietary Approach to Bulimia Treatment," *Physiology and Behavior* 33 (1984):769–75.

8. C. W. M. Wilson, "Clinical Pharmacologic Aspects of Ascorbic Acid," *Annals of the New York Academy of Sciences* 258 (1975):355–76. R. Hume and E. Weyers, "Changes in Leucocyte Ascorbic Acid During the Common Cold," *Scottish Medical Journal* 18 (1973):3–7. P. Roberts et al., "Vitamin C and Inflammation," *Medicine and Biology* 62 (1984):88–100.

9. W. R. Beisel, "Single Nutrients and Immunity," *American Journal of Clinical Nutrition* 35 (supplement) (1982):417–68. A. B. Carr et al., "Vitamin C and the Common Cold: Using Identical Twins as Controls," *Medical Journal of Australia* 2 (1981):411–12. J. Z. Miller et al., "Therapeutic Effect of Vitamin C: A Co-Twin Controlled Study," *Journal of the American Medical Association* 237 (1977):248–51.

10. L. E. Mansfield et al., "Food Allergy and Adult Migraine: Double-Blind and Mediator Confirmation of an Allergic Etiology," *Annals of Allergy* 55 (1985):126–31. J. Monro et al., "Migraine Is a Food-Allergic Disease," *Lancet* 2 (1984):719–21. J. Egger et al., "Is Migraine Food Allergy? A Double-Blind Controlled Trial of Oligoantigenic Diet Treatment," *Lancet* 2 (1983):865–69.

11. B. M. Altura, "Calcium Antagonist Properties of Magnesium: Implications for Anti-Migraine Actions," *Magnesium* 4 (1985):169–75.

12. McCarrent et al., "Amelioration of Severe Migraine by Fish Oil (N-3) Fatty Acids," *American Journal of Clinical Nutrition* 41 (Abstracts) (1985):874.

13. H. Bueno and L. Parrish, "The Bueno-Parrish Method (BPM) for Diagnosis of Intestinal Protozoa," *American Journal of Proctocology, Gastroenterology and Colon and Rectal Surgery* 32 (1981):6, 28.

14. M. Petitpierre et al., "Irritable Bowel Syndrome and Hypersensitivity to Food," *Annals of Allergy* 54 (1985):538–40. M. A. Smith et al., "Food Intolerance Atopy and Irritable Bowel Syndrome," *Lancet* 2 (1985):1064–66. R. Finn et al., "Expanding Horizons of Allergy and the Total Allergy Syndrome," *Clinical Ecology* 3 (1985):129–31. V. A. Alun-Jones et al., "Food Intolerance: A Major Factor in the Pathogenesis of Irritable Bowel Syndrome," *Lancet* 2 (1982):1115–17. J. Siegel, "Inflammatory Bowel Disease: Another Possible Facet of the Allergic Diathesis," *Annals of Allergy* 47 (1981):92–94.

15. D. Ratner et al., "Milk Protein–Free Diet for Nonseasonal Asthma and Migraine in Lactase-Deficient Patients," *Israel Journal of Medical Sciences* 19 (1983):806–809.

16. S. Schoenthaler, "Diet and Crime: An Empirical Examination of the Value of Nutrition in the Control and Treatment of Incarcerated Juvenile Offenders," *International Journal of Biosocial Research* 4 (1983):25–39. S. Schoenthaler and W. Doraz, "Types of Offenses Which Can Be Reduced in an Institutional Setting Using Nutritional Intervention: A Preliminary Empirical Evaluation," *International Journal of Biosocial Research* 4 (1983):74–84. S. Schoenthaler, "The Los Angeles Probation Department Diet-Behavior Program: An Empirical Evaluation of Six Institutions," *International Journal of Biosocial Research* 5 (1983):88–98. S. Schoenthaler, "The Northern California Diet-Behavior Program: An Empirical Examination of 3,000 Incarcerated Juveniles in Stanislaus County Juvenile Hall," *International Journal of Biosocial Research* 5 (1983):99–106. S. Schoenthaler, "The Alabama Diet-Behavior Program: An Empirical Evaluation at the Coosa Valley Regional Detention Center," *International Journal of Biosocial Research* 5 (1983):79–87.

17. D. S. King, "Can Allergic Exposure Provoke Psychological Symptoms?: A Double-Blind Test," *Biological Psychiatry* 16 (1981):3–17.

CHAPTER 9: HOW POWER-PACKED NUTRITION CREATES IMMUNITY FOR LIFE

1. M. Alter et al., "Diet and Multiple Sclerosis," *Archives of Neurology* 31 (1970):267–70.

2. R. L. Swank, "Multiple Sclerosis: 20 Years on a Low-Fat Diet," *Archives of Neurology* 23 (1970):460–74.

3. Z. Lucas and L. Power, "Dietary Fat Aggravates Active Rheumatoid Arthritis," *Clinical Research* 29 (1981):754a. L. Skoldstam, "Fasting and Vegan Diet in Rheumatoid Arthritis," *Scandinavian Journal of Rheumatology* 15 (1987):219–21.

4. R. H. Dworkin et al., "Linoleic Acid and Multiple Sclerosis: A Reanalysis of Three Double-Blind Trials," *Neurology* 34 (1984):1441–45. R. H. Dworkin, "Linoleic Acid and Multiple Sclerosis," *Lancet* 1 (1981):1153–54.

5. J. M. Kremer et al., "Effect of Manipulation of Dietary Fatty Acids on Clinical Manifestations of Rheumatoid Arthritis," *Lancet* 1 (1985):184–87. J. M. Kremer et al., "Fish Oil Fatty Acid Supplementation in Active Rheumatoid Arthritis: A Double-Blinded Crossover Study," *Annals of Internal Medicine* 106 (1987):497–503.

6. T. H. Lee et al., "Effect of Dietary Enrichment with Eicosapentaenoic and Docosahexaenoic Acids on *in Vitro* Neutrophile and Monocyte Leukotriene Synthesis in Rheumatoid Arthritis," *New England Journal of Medicine* 312 (1985):1217–24.

7. See Note 4 in this chapter.

8. D. R. Robinson et al., "The Protective Effect of Dietary Fish Oil on Murine Lupus," *Prostaglandins* 30 (1985):51–75. W. Yumura et al., "Dietary Fat and Immune Function—II. Effects on Immune Complex Nephritis (NZB x NZW) F_1 Mice," *Journal of Immunology* 136 (1985):3864–68. V. E. Kelley et al., "A Fish Oil Diet Rich in Eicosapentaenoic Acid Reduces Cyclooxygenase Metabolites and Suppresses Lupus in MRL-lpr Mice," *Journal of Immunology* 134 (1985):1949–59. D. G. Godfrey et al., "Effects of Dietary Supplementation on Autoimmunity in the MRL/lpr Mouse: A Preliminary Investigation," *Annals of the Rheumatic Diseases* 45 (1986):1019–24. D. Robinson et al., "Dietary Fish Oil Reduces Progression of Established Renal Disease (NZB x NZW) F_1 Mice and Delays Renal Disease in BXSB and MRL/l Strains," *Arthritis and Rheumatism* 29 (1986):539–49.

9. V. Johannson et al., "Nutritional Status in Girls with Juvenile Chronic Arthritis," *Human Nutrition: Clinical Nutrition* 40c (1986):57–67. U. Tarp et al., "Low Selenium Level in Severe Rheumatoid Arthritis," *Scandinavian Journal of Rheumatology* 14 (1987):97–100.

10. D. E. Mills and R. P. Ward, "Effects of Essential Fatty Acid Administration on Cardiovascular Responses to Stress in the Rat," *Lipids* 21 (1986):139–42. Kromhoudt et al., "The Inverse

Relationship Between Fish Consumption and 20-Year Mortality from Coronary Heart Disease," *New England Journal of Medicine* 312 (1985):1205–1209. B. E. Phillipson et al., "Reduction of Plasma Lipids, Lipoproteins, and Apoproteins by Dietary Fish Oils in Adults with Hyperlipidemia," *New England Journal of Medicine* 312 (1985):1210–16. P. G. Norris et al., "Effect of Dietary Supplementation with Fish Oil on Systolic Blood Pressure in Mild Essential Hypertension," *British Medical Journal* 293 (1986):104–105. J. Iacono et al., "Dietary Fats and the Management of Hypertension," *Canadian Journal of Physiology and Pharmacology* 64 (1986):856–62. P. Singer et al., "Blood Pressure- and Lipid-Lowering Effect of Mackerel and Herring Diet in Patients with Mild Essential Hypertension," *Atherosclerosis* 56 (1985):223–35.

11. Y. Rayssiguier and E. Gueux, "Magnesium and Lipids in Cardiovascular Disease," *Journal of the American College of Nutrition* 5 (1986):507–19.

12. H.-G. Classen, "Systemic Stress Magnesium Status and Cardiovascular Damage," *Magnesium* 5 (1986):105–10.

13. Kromhoudt et al., "Dietary Fiber and Ten-Year Mortality from Coronary Heart Disease, Cancer, and All Causes: The Zutphen Study," *Lancet* 2 (1982):518–22.

14. J. T. Salonen et al., "Association Between Cardiovascular Death and Myocardial Infarction and Serum Selenium in a Matched-Pair Longitudinal Study," *Lancet* 2 (1982):175–79.

15. D. P. Rose et al., "International Comparisons of Mortality Rates from Cancer of the Breast, Ovary, Prostate, and Colon and Per Capita Food Consumption," *Cancer* 54 (1986):2363–71.

16. R. A. Karmali, "Fatty Acids: Inhibition of Tumorigenesis," *American Journal of Clinical Nutrition* 45 (1987):225–29. H. Gabor and S. Abraham, "Effect of Dietary Menhaden Oil on Tumor Cell Loss and the Accumulation of Mass of a Transplantable Mammary Adenocarcinoma in Mice," *Journal of the National Cancer Institute* 76 (1986):1223–29. J. J. Jurkowski and W. T. Cave, Jr., "Dietary Effects of Menhaden Oil on the Growth and Membrane Lipid Composition of Rat Mammary Tumors," *Journal of the National Cancer Institute* 74 (1985):1145–50. B. S. Reddy and H. Maruyama, "Effect of Dietary Fish Oil on Azoxymethane-Induced Colon Carcinogenesis in Male F344 Rats," *Cancer Research* 46 (1986):3367–70.

17. D. P. Burkitt et al., "Dietary Fiber and Disease," *Journal of the American Medical Association* 229 (1974):1068–73.

18. See Note 13 in this chapter.

19. "Micronutrient Interactions in the Prevention of Cancer," *Nutrition Reviews* 45 (1987):139–40. W. C. Willett et al., "Prediagnostic Serum Selenium and Risk of Cancer," *Lancet* 1 (1983):130–34. M. S. Menkes et al., "Serum Beta-Carotene, Vitamins A and E, Selenium, and the Risk of Lung Cancer," *New England Journal of Medicine* 315 (1986):1250–54. J. T. Salonen et al., "Risk of Cancer in Relation to Serum Concentrations of Selenium and Vitamins A and E: Matched Case Control Analysis of Prospective Data," *British Medical Journal* 290 (1985):417–20.

Index